Kilfillan House
A Haven of Care

Julian Ashbourn

Copyright © 2017 Julian Ashbourn
All Rights Reserved
ISBN: 1975805968
ISBN -13: 978-1975805968

This book is dedicated to all those who act as carers and nurses within care homes throughout Britain. It is a demanding and often stressful job, with long hours, caring for those who, for whatever reason, need a little help. For many patients, it is their last stop on the journey of life and it is impossible not to feel for them accordingly. This renders the already hard work of carers quite poignant, and they have to deal with situations that most of us do not face within our own occupations. Their dedication and humanity is essential to the operation of these sanctuaries among the hubbub of modern life. No praise is too high for these individuals, without whom, our world would certainly be a poorer place.

Contents

1	Introduction	Page 1
2	A Brief History of Kilfillan House	Page 2
3	The Gardens	Page 6
4	The House	Page 14
5	The Staff	Page 22
6	The Residents	Page 30
7	Reflections	Page 34

1 Introduction

This is the story of Kilfillan House, a Bupa Care Home situated in a quite road in Berkhamsted in Hertfordshire. In many respects, it is, no doubt, like many other such care homes along the length and breadth of Britain. Its staff come in day after day and night after night to care for a group of patients who will, themselves, be resident every day. The patient's condition will vary between those who remain physically active and who maintain an interest in things in general, and those who, alas, are bedridden and need almost constant care. Many have dementia and other conditions which are particularly trying on occasion. And then, some of them pass and, of a sudden, are residents no more. The carers and nurses must take all of this in their stride and continue as though they are not affected by such things, although, of course they must be affected to one degree or another.

But why produce a book about care homes at all? Surely, everyone is aware of them and what part they play within our broader social architecture? Certainly, those who have close relatives in care homes will know about them, although, even they will typically only experience a certain aspect of the home. And so, this book will open up care homes in such a manner as the reader might understand the work and dedication which goes on within the walls of a typical care home. In addition, it celebrates a particular institution, Kilfillan House, a Bupa Care Home in Berkhamsted, which has served the local community for many years. It is indeed a sanctuary, where individuals in need come to rest and be cared for by the staff.

The reader will be taken on a tour of Kilfillan House and its grounds and will be introduced to the workings of such an institution. They will come to understand what a care home actually does and why we need them within the community.

2 A Brief History of Kilfillan House

Berkhamsted used to be a lovely old Market Town, like many in Britain, where farmers and traders would meet together and all manner of produce could be bought. But Berkhamsted has been around for a long time. It is where, in December 1066, William the Conqueror took possession of England, by which time, people had already been living in the area for a very long time. In fact, evidence of flint working in the Neolithic period has been found, together with indications of metal working, later in the Iron Age. It seems that the particular siting of Berkhamsted, within the Bulbourne Valley, at the end of the Chilterns, has attracted settlers for around 5000 years. Berkhamsted High Street was known by the Saxons as Akeman Street and was on a major route, even before the Romans came.

The earliest written reference to Berkhamsted was in 970 AD and, in 1086, it was recorded in the Domesday Book as an ancient borough. Berkhamsted Castle flourished between 1066 and 1495, when it was a favoured spot for many royals and nobility when travelling through, or even staying for some considerable time. After 1495, the town seemed to go into decline and the Castle fell into disuse, eventually being partly dismantled, no doubt in support of other building projects. However, with the coming of the canals and the railways in the 19th century, Berkhamsted became once more a thriving town on the main route from London right up to the Midlands and beyond. Imagine the bustle, with barges coming up and down the canal and moving through the locks, while horse-drawn carriages of all types clattered through the high street, to and from the surrounding farms and main areas of residence and business. By 1835 there were a great many residential houses, with a fair proportion of what were described as 'handsome residences' as more influential people moved into the area. By 1887, the population of Berkhamsted had been recorded at 4,485.

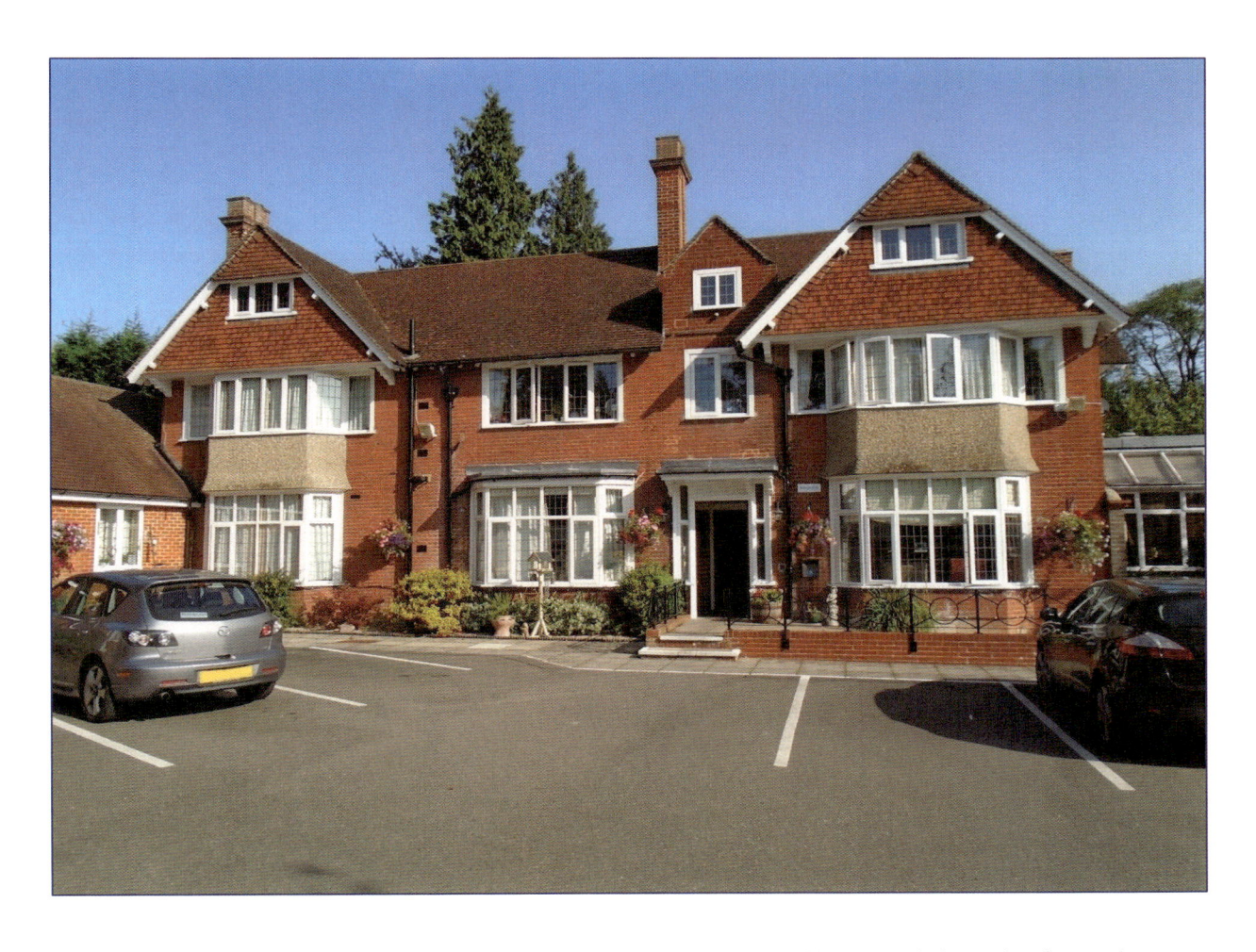

Kilfillan House as it is today, bathed by sunshine on a hot Berkhamsted day. The front door is open and visitors may come and go freely.

And so, Berkhamsted was becoming a thriving town which already had a distinguished history behind it. The school had existed since the 16th century and had produced many notable individuals, and the town had grown steadily. However, it remained surrounded by fields and farms and, having populated the High Street and immediately surrounding areas, prospective residents sought to stretch their wings a little and build desirable residences further up on the hill. In 1877, the site which would eventually bear Kilfillan House was itself a field. Field no. 318 in fact, according to the Ordnance Survey. Graemesdyke Road had yet to be built and everywhere was green and buzzing with nature. But the field was bought and sold and, eventually, in 1907, the land fell into the hands of Charlotte Boyd and work soon started on laying out the extensive plot, which stretched right up to what is now Cross Oak Road and extended a fair distance northward. The house was built and, originally, had lovely gardens which were especially landscaped. It must, in those early years, have been a most beautiful place to live, with views down towards the town, and southward into the valley, although other large houses would soon appear as Graemesdyke Road became a desirable area in which to live.

Strange things happen within the lifetime of a house and, in 1932, Kilfillan House became an asset of the Chesham Electric Light and Power Company. In 1947, the myriad of private electricity companies were nationalized and the Chesham Electric Light and Power Company was merged, with many others, into the Eastern Electricity Board. In 1950, Edith Millen came along and a change of use was granted for Kilfillan House to become a school. The school was successful and ran along until 1968 when, sadly, the house was converted into a number of flats. Four years later, a third of the land was sold off and the Kilfillan House estate shrank considerably. Miss Millen finally passed away in 1986 and within two years, another third of the original land was sold off and Kilfillan House became a nursing home. The nursing home ran along nicely and, in 1997, it was acquired by Bupa who continued to run it as a nursing home, although, it is now designated as a care home. And so, dear old Kilfillan House has seen many changes, including to the other large homes in the area, many of which also sold off portions of their land for building purposes. But Kilfillan retains a certain charm of its own, although it is much altered from its original state.

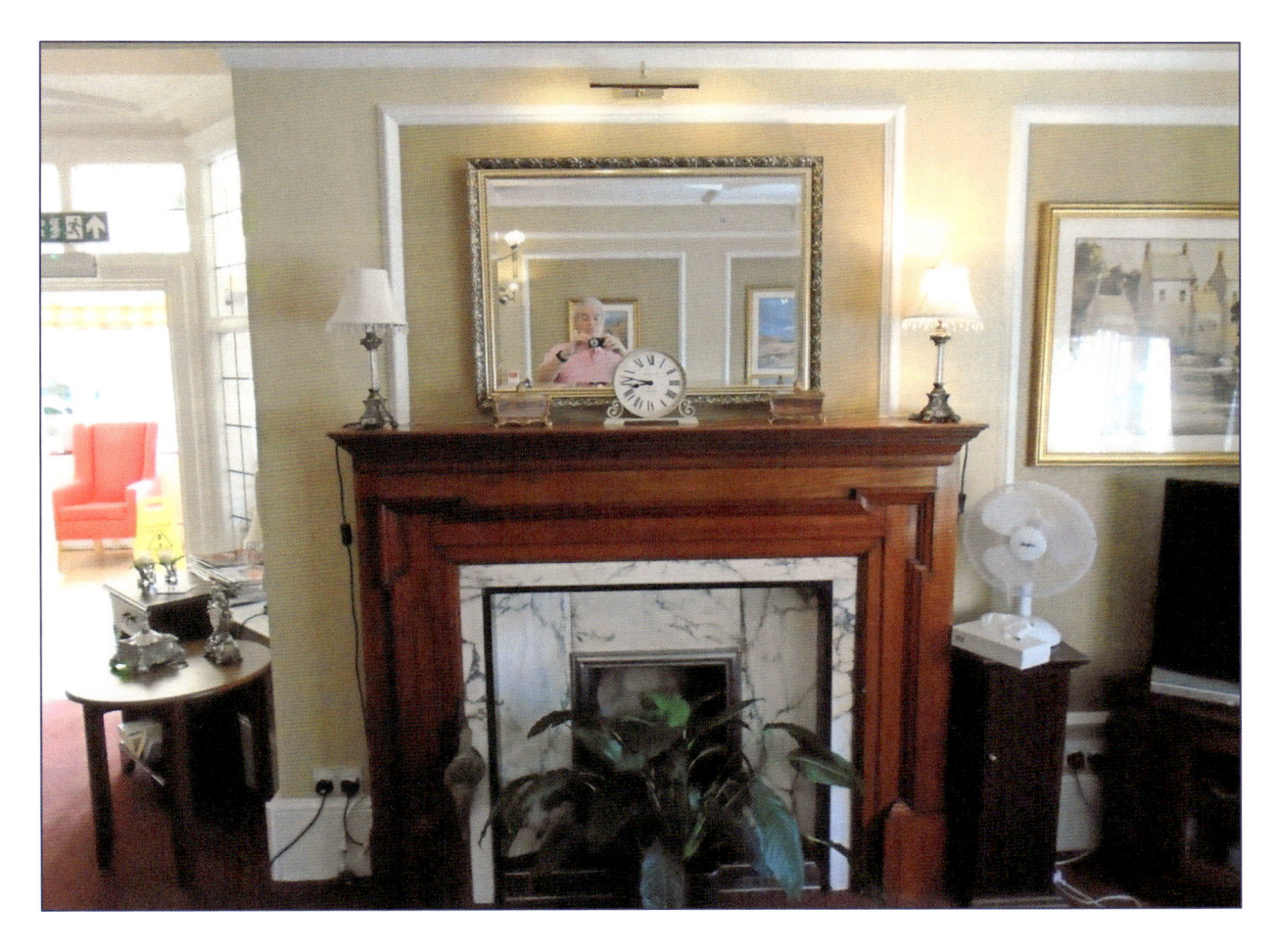

The fireplace in the lounge with its beautiful woodwork and inset granite finishing still looks homely and reassuring.

3 The Gardens

Of course, most of the original gardens are now houses, behind and on both sides of Kilfillan House, but it does retain a small garden area, together with a conservatory, and this is much appreciated by residents who like to walk in the garden for exercise, or, if they are wheelchair bound, they may still sit out in the garden on a warm day and enjoy the scene of nature all around them.

The gardens are very well tended in Kilfillan House, by one of the staff members who keeps an eye on the garden throughout the year as the seasons bring their own variety of colour and temporary residents, such as birds and squirrels. Bees, wasps and ants are also quite busy at various times, and it is interesting to watch them interact with the various plants. There is usually a blaze of colour somewhere within the garden and, in the summer, the whole area is alight with the finest of Mother Nature's palette as a huge variety of plants come to life.

A garden is an important part of any home, but it is especially important for a Care Home. The opportunity, just to see a garden in bloom, is uplifting for the spirit when one is at a low ebb, as many residents are, from time to time. For those who are able, the pleasure of just sitting and reading in a secluded garden spot is invaluable as a part of their medical therapy. Furthermore, it is a wonderful place to welcome visitors, especially on a nice day when the sun is shining and there is a gentle breeze in the air. What could be more charming than sitting and having tea with your relatives in such a setting.

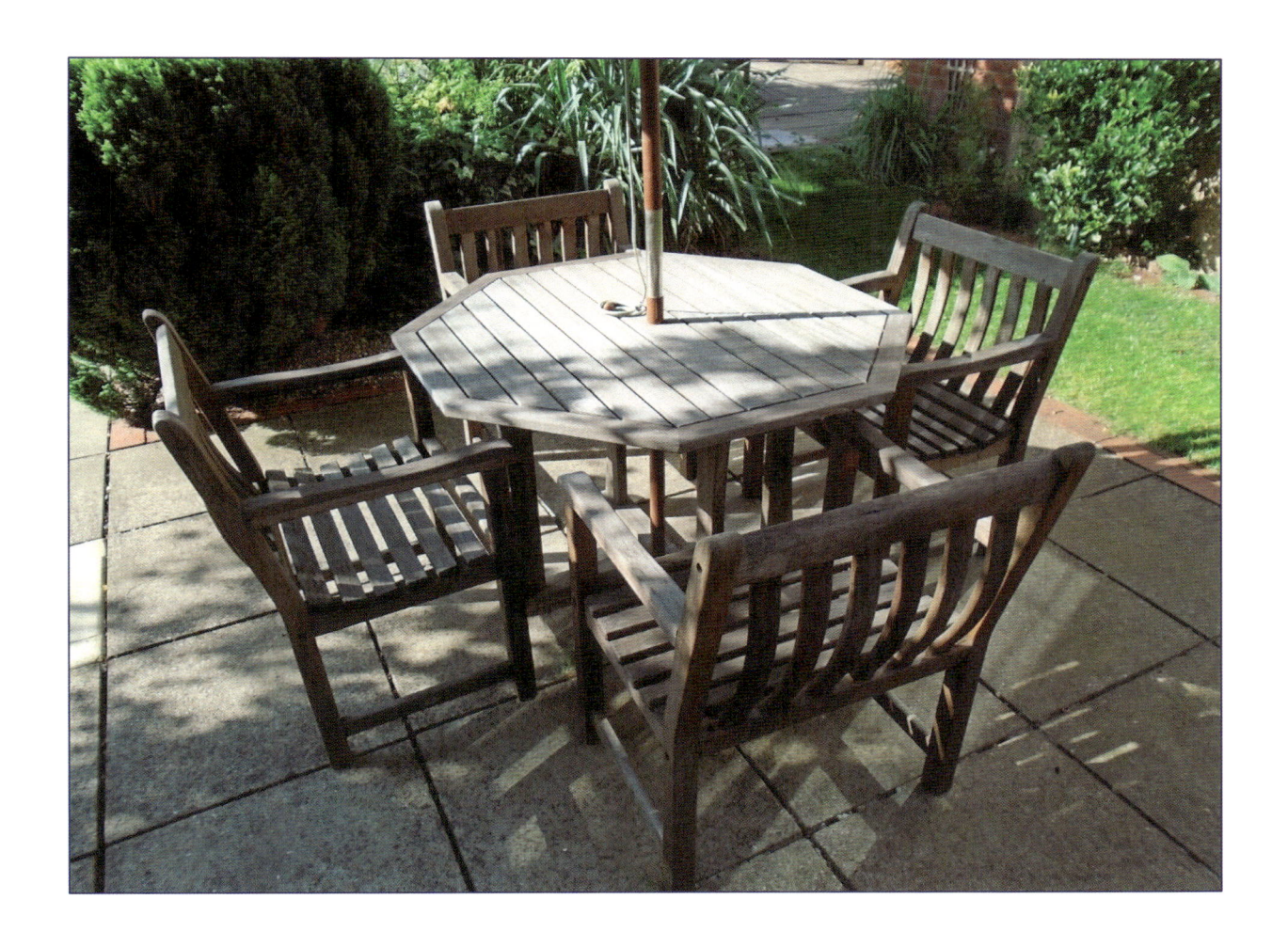

There are several nice tables and chairs at Kilfillan House, together with some separate benches at various locations throughout the gardens.

The gardens at Kilfillan House are lovingly tended by the staff and provide a cornucopia of flowers, resplendent in their coats of many colours and huge variety of forms. The closer you look, the more you will discover about the miracle of nature. Every little leaf, every part of every blossom, all exquisite in their design and execution. The bees like to hop from one flower to another and the occasional butterfly will pass by from time to time. Indeed, one is never alone and, depending upon the time of day, several wild birds may keep you company, interspersed by squirrels who, with their various antics, will keep you entertained for hours.

This reconnection with nature is, in fact, part of the therapy and affects the well-being of staff and patients alike, together with the wide array of visitors to Kilfillan House. It is inspiring in itself and reminds us how life always finds a way and, in doing so, produces the most amazing creations to be seen on our planet, albeit sometimes in miniature. The spectrum of colours that shine through on a sunny day are unlike those to be found on any artist's palette, and no artist could create a scene so beautiful. And yet, this beauty abounds in the little garden at Kilfillan, not just in the flowers, but in a variety of larger shrubs and trees. It also exists within the various insects to be found wandering around, some on the wing, and some on the ground, within the cracks in the paving stones and on the grass. Life puts on a wonderful display wherever you look.

It makes you wonder what the original gardens would have been like at Kilfillan House. We know that they were properly landscaped and, no doubt, they had a wonderful variety of shrubs and plants which would come alive in the spring and summer, with a subtly different set to greet tired eyes in the greyness of autumn and winter. Gardens were an important part of all great houses and, indeed, are an important part of our heritage. A garden, no matter how small, brings pleasure and a sense of calm to all who engage with it. The garden at Kilfillan House, although much smaller than the original is, consequently, very important indeed, for all the reasons given.

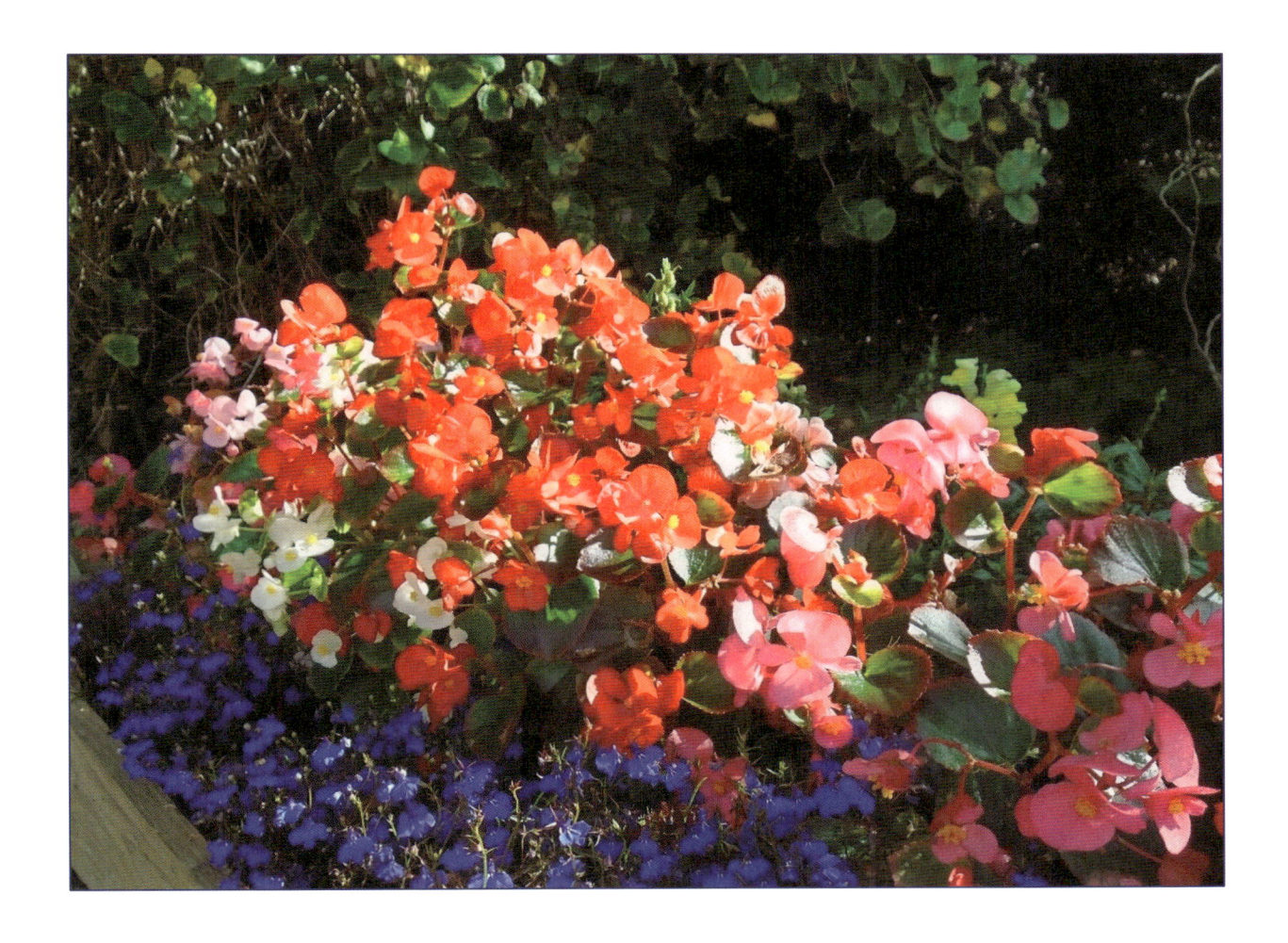

The range of colours and shapes, even within a small space, is quite astonishing. The garden at Kilfillan House is full of such surprises.

Here is a little verse about trees.

He stood as lonely as a tree
His gaze stretched out across the sea
To wonder whence we had begun
Our troubled race beneath the sun

The toil, the blood, the sweat and tears
Our broken dreams that mark the years
We once aspired to better things
Written large neath angels wings

Are we now bound forever more
To visualise the distant shores
Where Dolphins once played in the sea
And birds found shelter in the trees

We yearn for days in far off lands
With forests green, unspoiled by man
Where creatures great and creatures small
Would sing their songs in Nature's hall

In days of old we often spoke
Of chivalry and hearts of oak
But no human heart shall ever be
As pure and noble as a tree

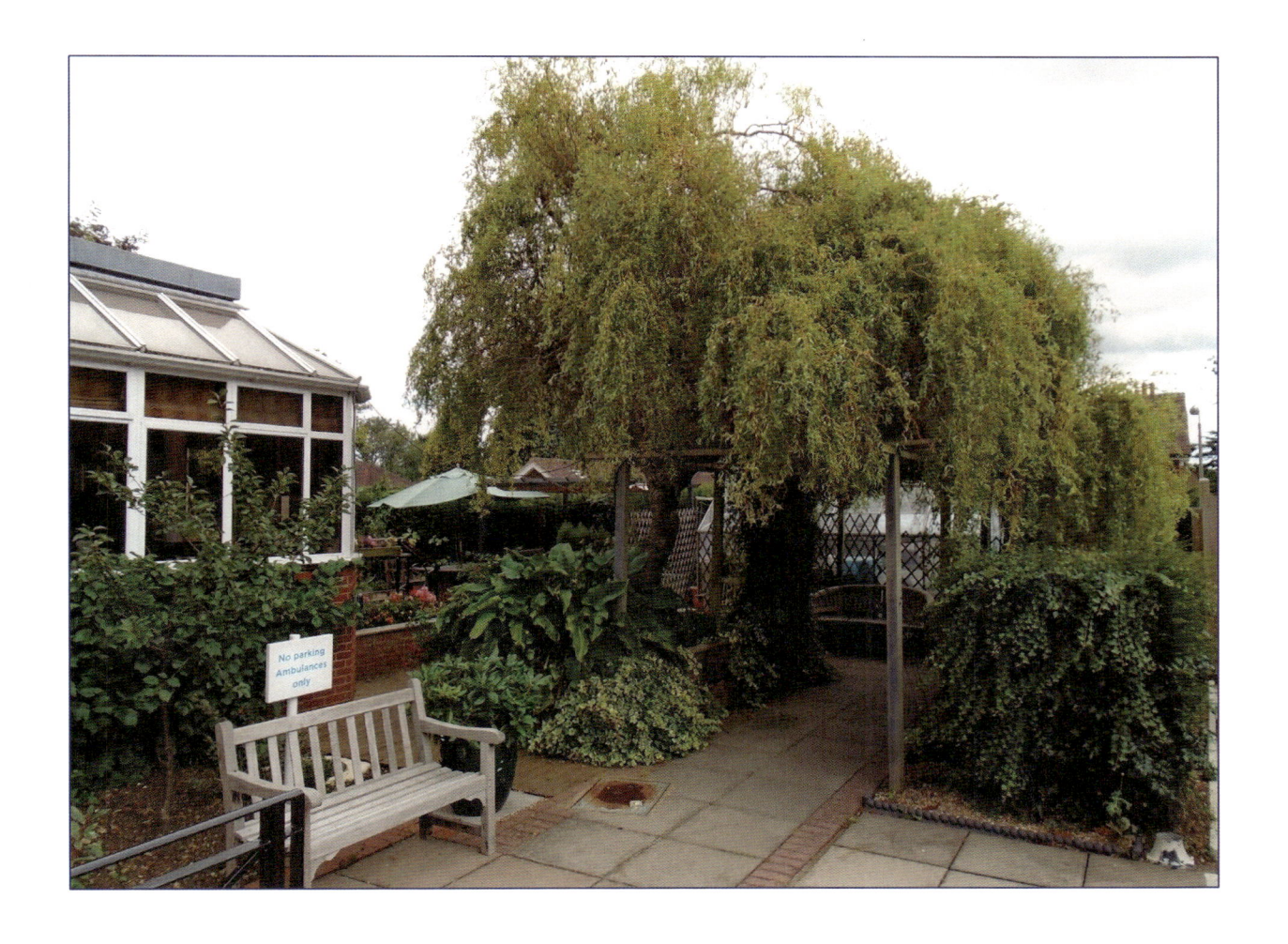

Here is a nice spot to sit and watch the world go by, as this particular seat faces forwards towards Graemsdyke Road.

Of course, if you have a garden, then you really should have a conservatory where people can sit on a cooler day and still enjoy the pleasures of the garden. Kilfillan House has a beautiful, large conservatory, which serves a number of purposes.

- Certainly, you can sit in the conservatory and still enjoy all the sights and sounds of the garden, and many do just that, especially when the weather is changeable or perhaps a little too breezy to be outside.
- The conservatory acts as a meeting place where patients often gather in the morning and are able to enjoy a chat and a cup of tea.
- It also serves as an activity room, and there are many such activities, some of which involve direct participation, such as various crafts, and some of which are group activities, such as quizzes, which are always very popular.
- The conservatory, at certain times of day, is also a quiet environment where you can sit and enjoy a good book. This is especially true of evenings.
- There is a widescreen television and a DVD player in the conservatory, enabling residents to watch their favourite films if desired.

There is much more to this versatile and lovely area of Kilfillan House and it often acts as the centre of activities.

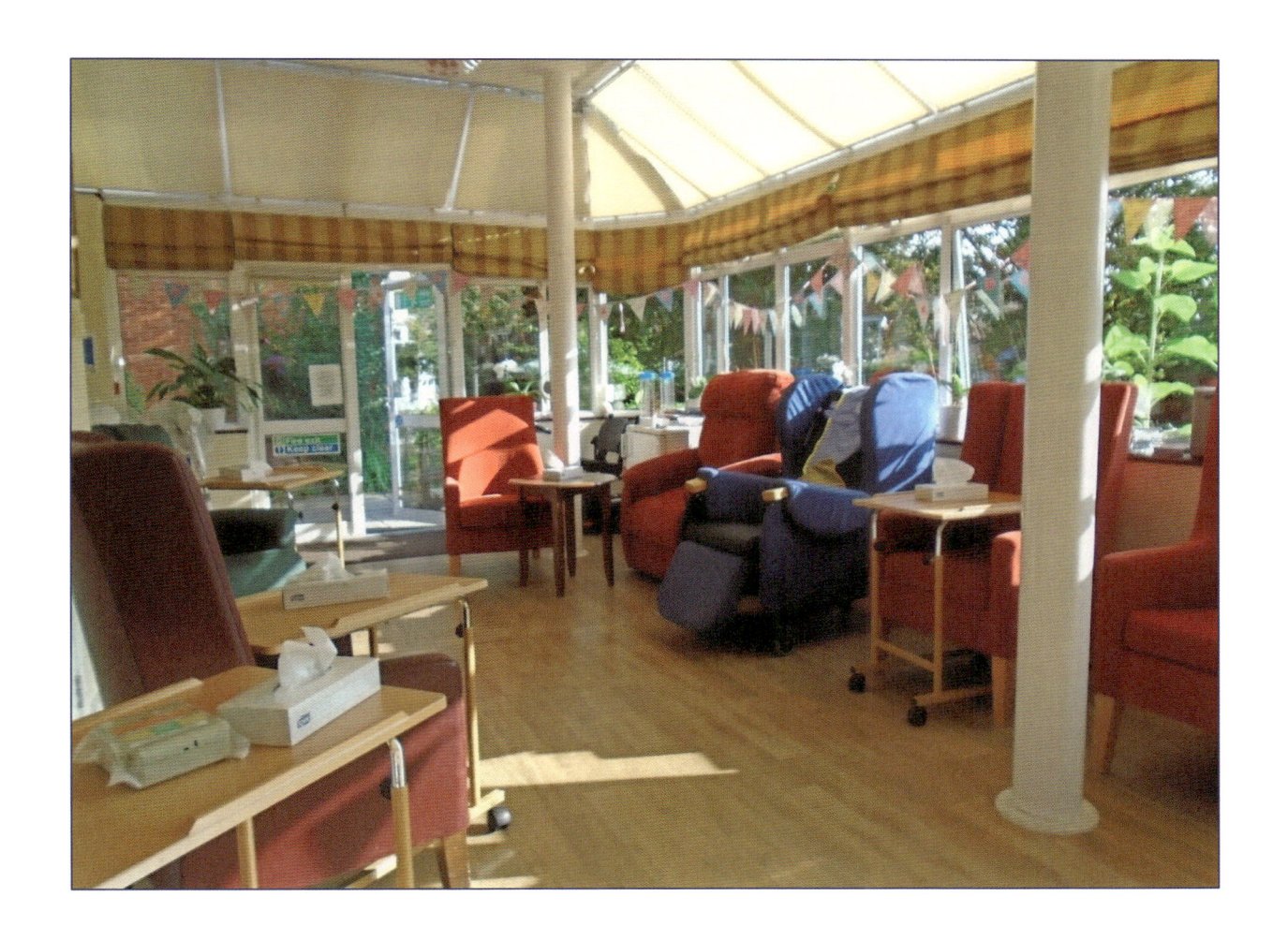

A view from inside the conservatory. This shot is taken from about two thirds down the length of the area. Behind us are more tables and a television screen.

4 The House

Kilfillan House itself is a lovely old, rambling building which retains some of its original wood cladding in the reception area and lounge. The rooms were originally all quite large but have since been restructured in order to accommodate individual care rooms. But still, coming down the broad stair-case into the reception area, you get a sense of what the house used to be like and what a lovely family home it must have been.

Architecturally, it is quite interesting, with sections seeming to but on to the main fabric of the building. To the rear, there is a continuation of the building line with a second building, which is not actually part of the Care Home, but a row of apartments for elderly folk or others with needs. There are many windows which look out over equally many vistas. Some of them quite interesting, when they overlook the garden or face towards the front of the house, and others rather less so. Nevertheless, it remains an interesting building and has a homely feel about it, which is conducive to its current function as a care home. For patients, this *is* their home and it is important that they can feel comfortable in it. Even for staff, they spend long hours here and it is, effectively, *their* second home.

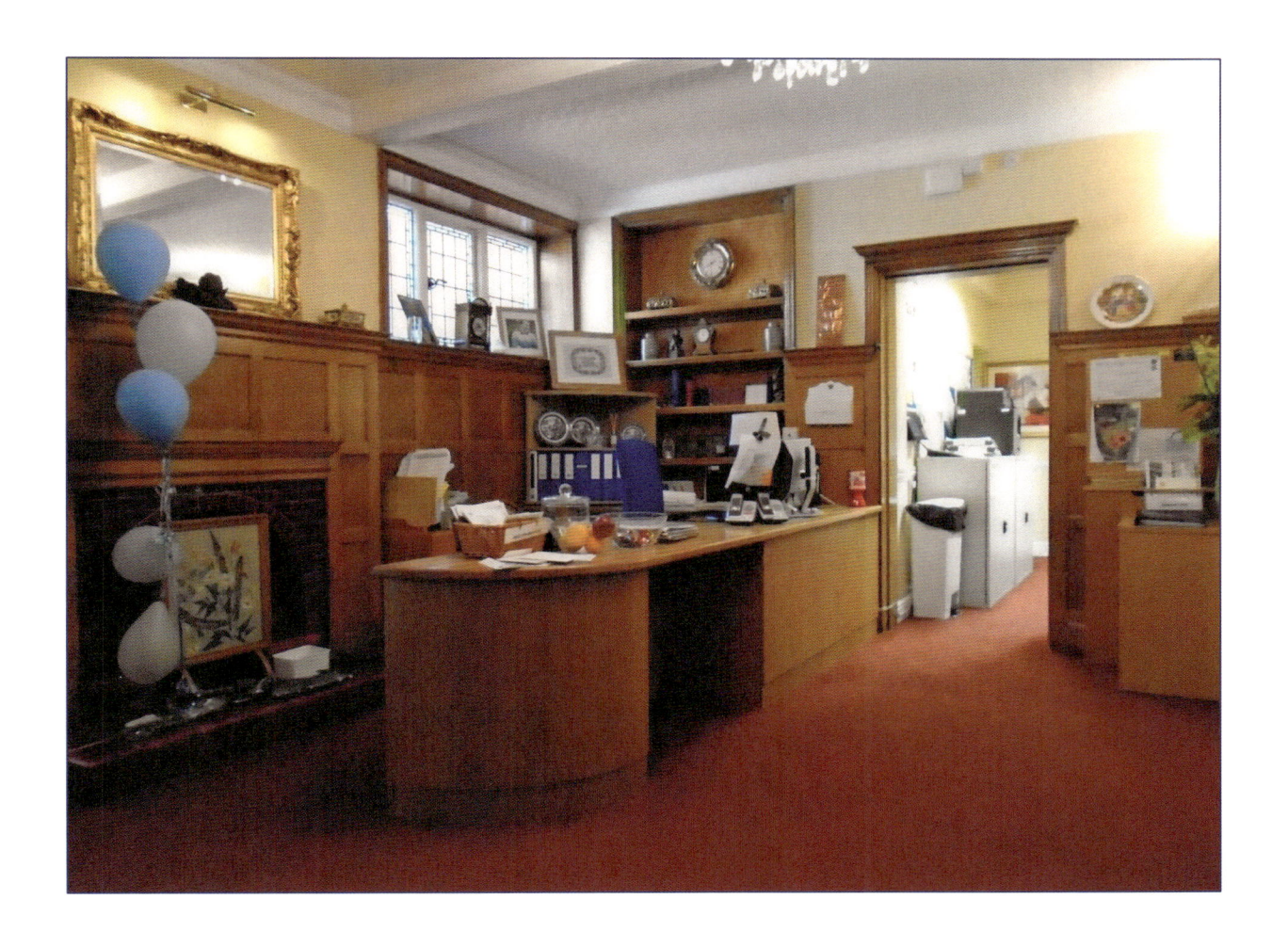

The Reception area provides a glimpse of what the whole of the house used to be like.

As a consequence of splitting the originally large rooms into smaller compartments for individual en-suite rooms, there are various hallways which lead off from the main stairwell area, both upstairs and downstairs. These lend an air of mystery to the house, especially for new residents. It also reminds everyone that, notwithstanding the conversion, it remains a house and a home. But a home is more than bricks and mortar and only comes alive when populated. The staff and patients at Kilfillan House are, in fact, the home, as they provide the human element which characterises the house itself. Their voices, individual characters, sounds and the never ceasing activity bring life into the walls, corridors and common areas, such as the lounge, the conservatory and the dining area. Indeed, Kilfillan House is bustling with activity throughout the day, when visitors are also welcome and there are often relatives to be found participating in various activities.

Visitors who simply wish to visit in order to understand how a Care Home functions are also welcome at any time, and there is always someone to show them around and explain the operation.

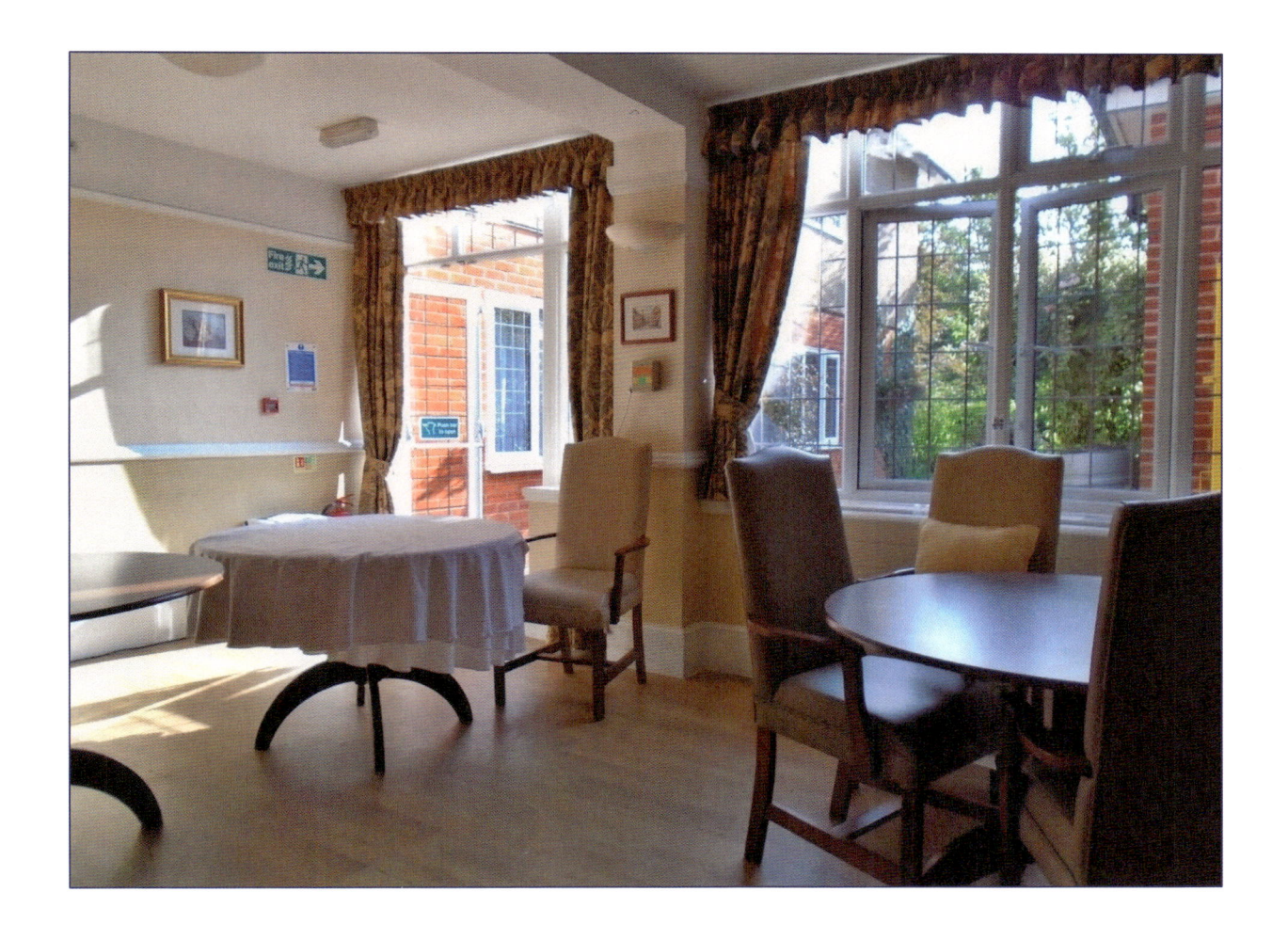

The dining area as it is being busily prepared for the next meal. Residents may also be served in their rooms if preferred.

And so, each day, Kilfillan House wakes up to a bustle of activity as breakfast is prepared and patients are given their medication, where applicable. This is a busy time as the nurses will also check the wellbeing of every patient and ensure that they are comfortable and ready for the day ahead. After breakfast, residents may decide where they would like to be and, very often, the conservatory is a popular choice. Those who cannot safely walk by themselves are brought by the carers in wheelchairs. The conservatory has a music system and so, if residents wish, they may listen to their favourite music, and there is a wide choice available from which to choose. On a dull morning, this tends to lift the spirits a little.

After a while, a tea and coffee trolley comes around, usually sporting some tasty cakes or chocolate éclairs or some such treat. Residents may like to chat with each other, or read, or just enjoy the moment. If it is a warm day, there are two sets of French windows which may be opened, together with opening windows along the side of the conservatory. If the sun is a little too strong, there are blinds which may be lowered accordingly. If preferred, residents may like to sit in the lounge and catch up with world events via the wide screen television which is usually switched on, or simply relax in the comfortable chairs provided for the purpose.

In any event, most residents are able to leave their rooms for a good part of the day. In their absence, their rooms will be cleaned and the beds changed and made up ready for the evening. Those residents who are unable to leave their rooms will be tended to by the nurses and carers and made as comfortable as possible. This is the very essence of a Care Home, to ensure that every resident is attended to throughout the day, and night as well, if necessary.

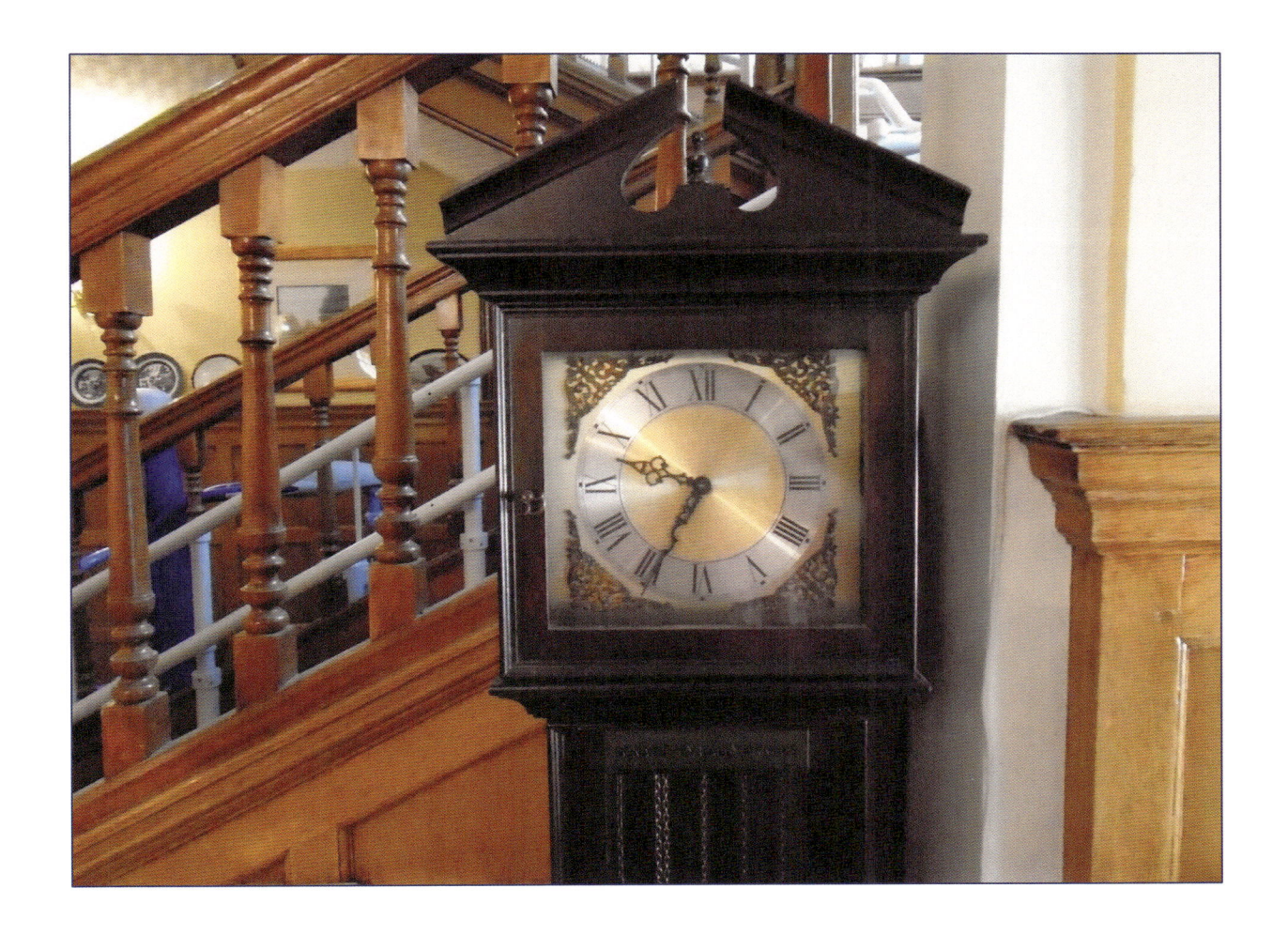

There is always something occurring at Kilfillan House, as the grandfather clock winds its way slowly around the dial and chimes out its messages.

The walls of Kilfillan House contain a world within a world. They have been host to a family home, a school, and now a Care Home. The word 'sanctuary' used in the title of this book is apt, as the house is indeed a sanctuary for residents, away from the cares of the world, and yet, still in touch with local and broader activities, to whatever degree they wish. Visitors and relatives bring news of family affairs, but otherwise, Kilfillan is its own little community, bustling with its own affairs, as it has done since it was originally built.

For residents, Kilfillan House is their home. They live here and are a key component of the house and its activities. For some, it may prove to be their final resting place on this Earth, and so it is important that the sense of 'home' prevails at all times. This is aided by the staff who become part of the resident's family. Being with them every day and befriending them accordingly. It is a dynamic family which grows as relatives and visitors become familiar with the house and those who live here.

There is a good deal of entertainment provided by visiting professionals, who always lift the spirits with their songs and banter. Some of them are surprisingly good and all of them interesting in one way or another. Residents are also welcome to engage in a number of group activities from quizzes to arts and crafts and these are always well received. Alternatively, residents may become involved in their own little projects (such as this book for example) in order to remain constructive, in spite of their particular illness or condition.

And so, the walls of Kilfillan House reverberate to a life of its own. A world where management, nurses and carers come together with a wide spectrum of residents, each of whom have their own fascinating story, and each of whom contribute to the community which constitutes the Care Home. For Care Homes are indeed a community apart, with many strands that come together to form the whole.

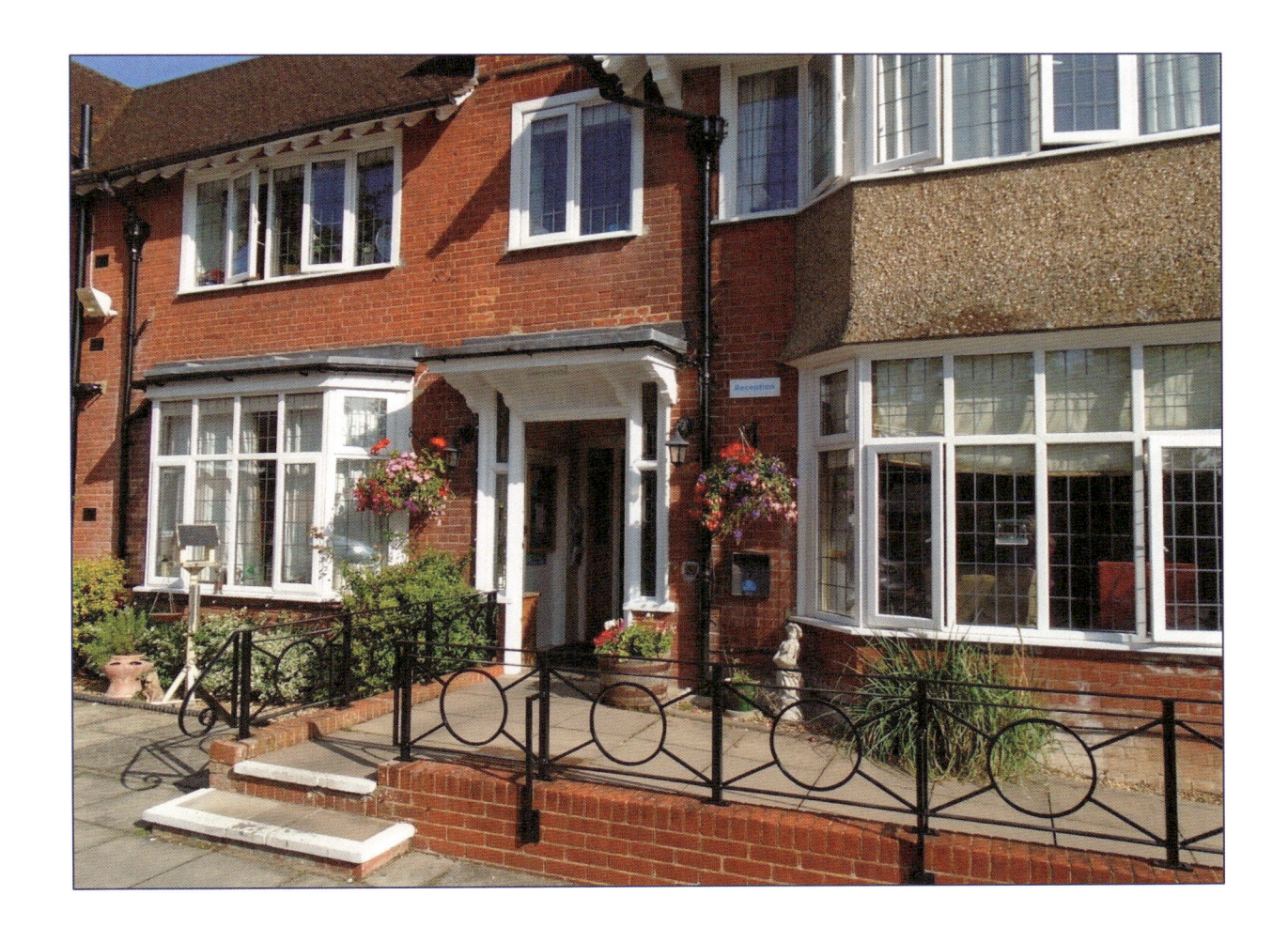

The welcoming front door of Kilfillan House, through which many have passed in the history of this most interesting building.

5 The Staff

The staff play a vitally important role in the day to day life of Kilfillan House. They are the engine that powers the ship and without which it would be meaningless. They are also the visible interface between the organisation that runs the care home and those who are resident there, together with their visiting relations.

The staff should therefore embody the ethics and methodology employed by the organisation responsible for the smooth running of the facility. But more than this, they should be able to interface with the residents on a practical, day to day basis. They should become 'family' as far as the residents are concerned, for the are the only day by day family that the residents may enjoy. Furthermore, it is considerably more pleasant and inspiring for the staff to have this close interaction and involvement with the residents. Like all relationships, these can take a little time to form properly, but they are the very core of a successful Care Home.

Consequently, caring for residents at a Care Home is a job like no other. Naturally, it involves a certain degree of routine and expertise, but it also involves the creation of a web of special relationships with residents, that simply doesn't occur in the majority of professions. It takes a very special person to undertake this role. A role for which the rewards include the aforementioned relationships, some of which may become quite complex.

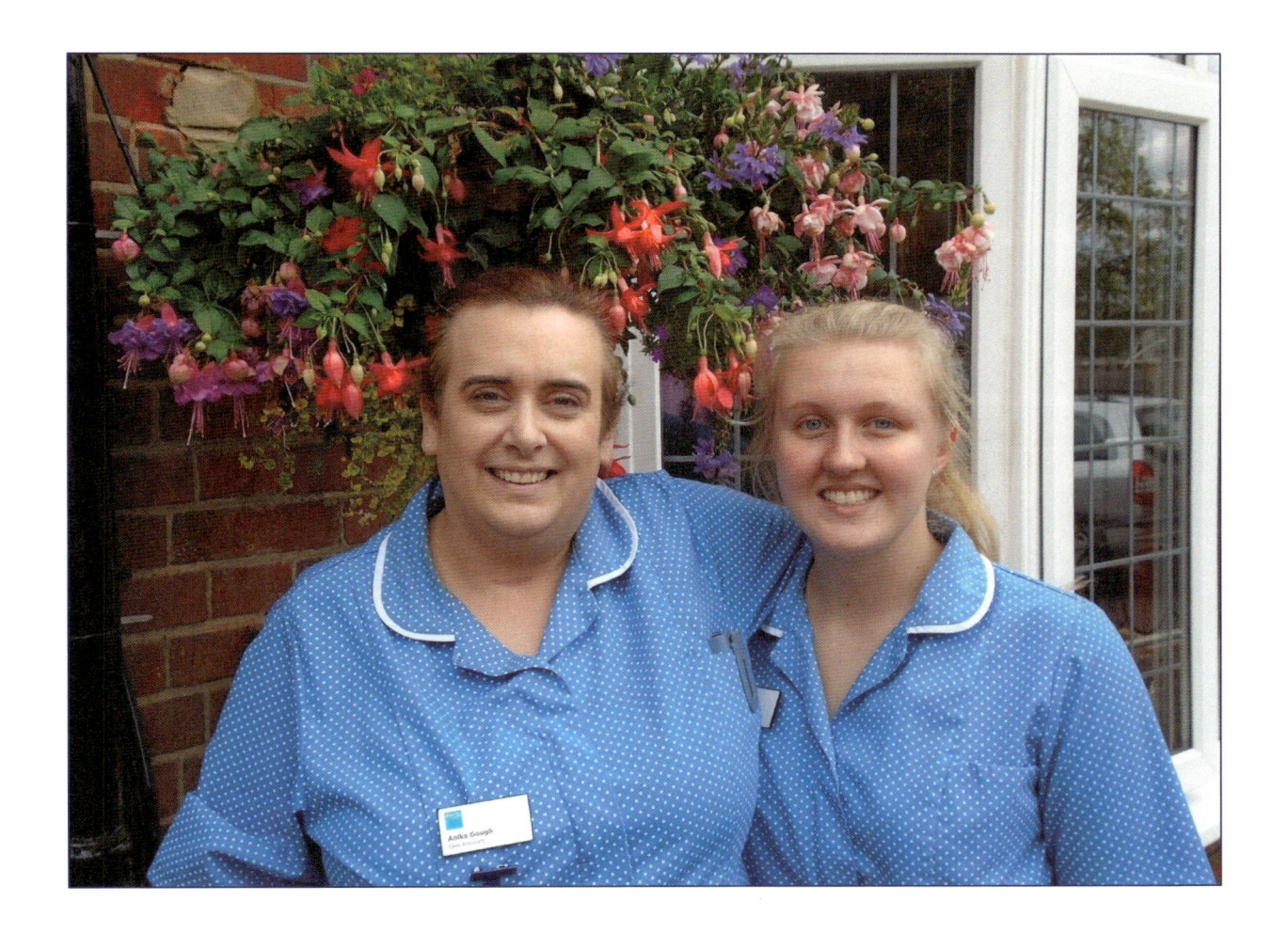

It takes a very special person to assume the role of a carer or nurse at a Care Home.

For the resident, the carer is their immediate lifeline. The carer is their friend and confidante to whom they may express their feelings and ideas from day to day. The carer also takes care of their immediate needs, such as preparing their bed, bringing them a nice cup of tea when required, or simply sitting with them for a much needed chat. The carer will also notice any slight change in the resident's condition and notify an on duty nurse where appropriate, in order to check that everything is as it should be.

The nurse, in turn, is responsible for dispensing medication, according to a very precisely defined chart for each patient. Some of these medications will necessarily be quite strong and the nurses are therefore responsible for their security. This is usually achieved via storage within a robust, locked cabinet, which is taken from room to room as required. There is also a strict timetable to be adhered to, and this may be different for each patient.

In addition to these duties, the nurses must check the overall wellbeing of each resident and, upon noticing any significant change, will need to notify the doctor, under which that particular resident is registered. That doctor may, in turn, consult with specialist doctors according to the precise illness, or set of illnesses, suffered by the resident. In such a manner, a programme of medical care may be constructed and tailored for each resident. Consequently, there may be many behind the scenes discussions and consultations that occur on behalf of the resident, the objective being to provide suitable treatment and ensure that they are as comfortable as possible.

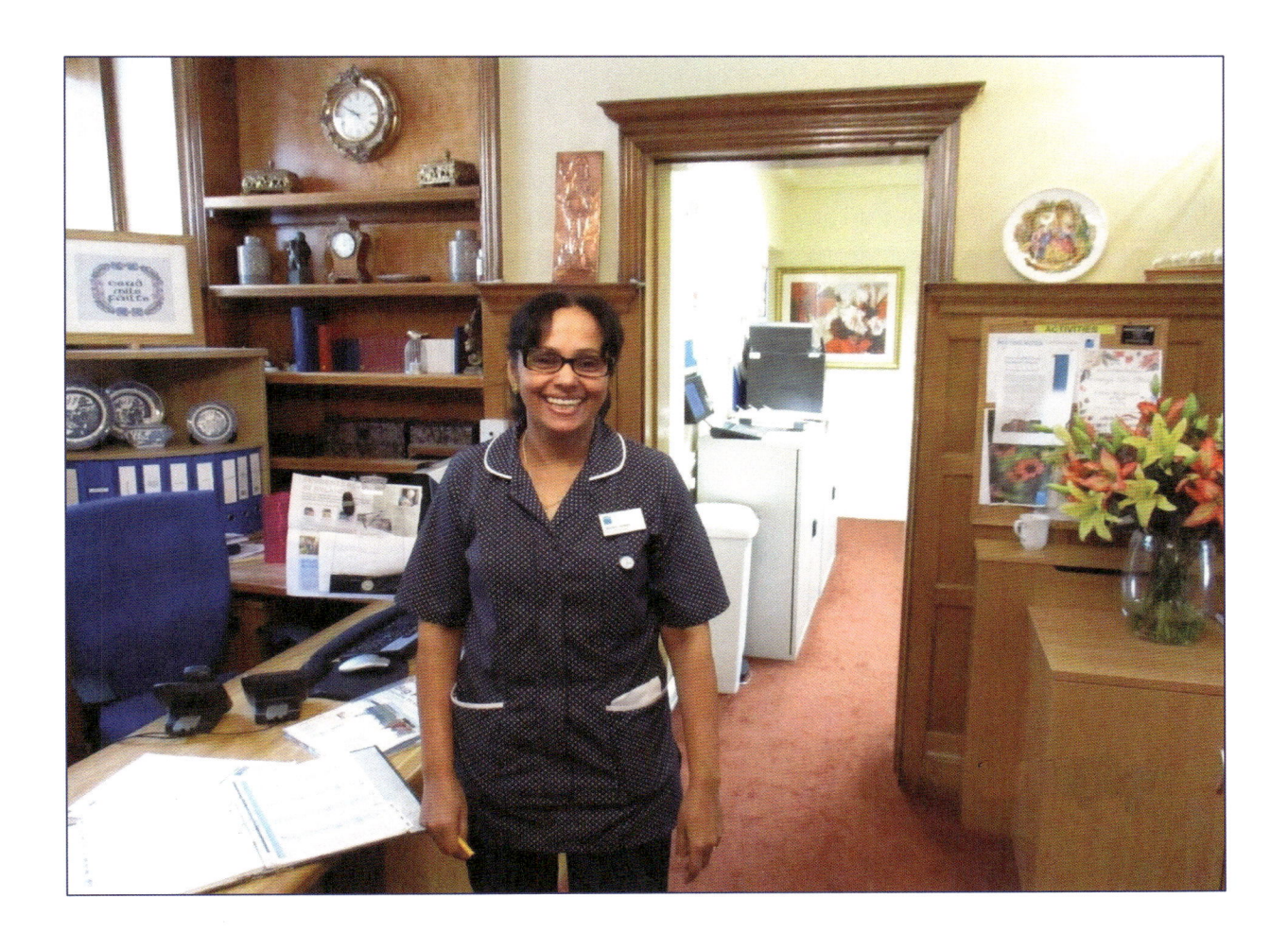

The nurses job is complex and must necessarily embrace many factors including, of course, the overall welfare of the resident.

These functions of carer and nurse are pivotal within a Care Home. However, there are other functions, some of them behind the scenes, that make up the machinery of care. Among these are the managerial functions which keep the Care Home operating according to a defined set of standards. These managerial functions can be very time consuming and exacting in their execution. They include managing the supply chain, for all the materials and consumables required for everyday operation. Then there is the acquisition of all necessary drugs and medications which must be available round the clock, including those that might be utilized under emergency conditions.

In addition to the managerial function, there are the housekeeping functions which include cleaning, laundry and other such basic requirements. Then there are the kitchen functions and cooking for a large number of residents, some of whom may have special dietary requirements, together with the necessary clearing and cleaning tasks. The Care Home is rather like a hotel in this context and must be managed accordingly.

Then there is the maintenance of the facility itself to consider. Some of this may be undertaken by an onboard 'maintenance man', at least for the everyday minor repairs and the replacement of consumables. Other tasks will require specialist teams to be called in and managed accordingly. All of this must be allowed for within a managed budget, and so, financial management must also form a part of the overall management task. In short, there is a great deal of behind the scenes activity inherent in the running of a successful Care Home. However, it is the carers and nurses who really define the character of the establishment, and their roles are crucial within the overall kaleidoscope of factors which constitute the facility.

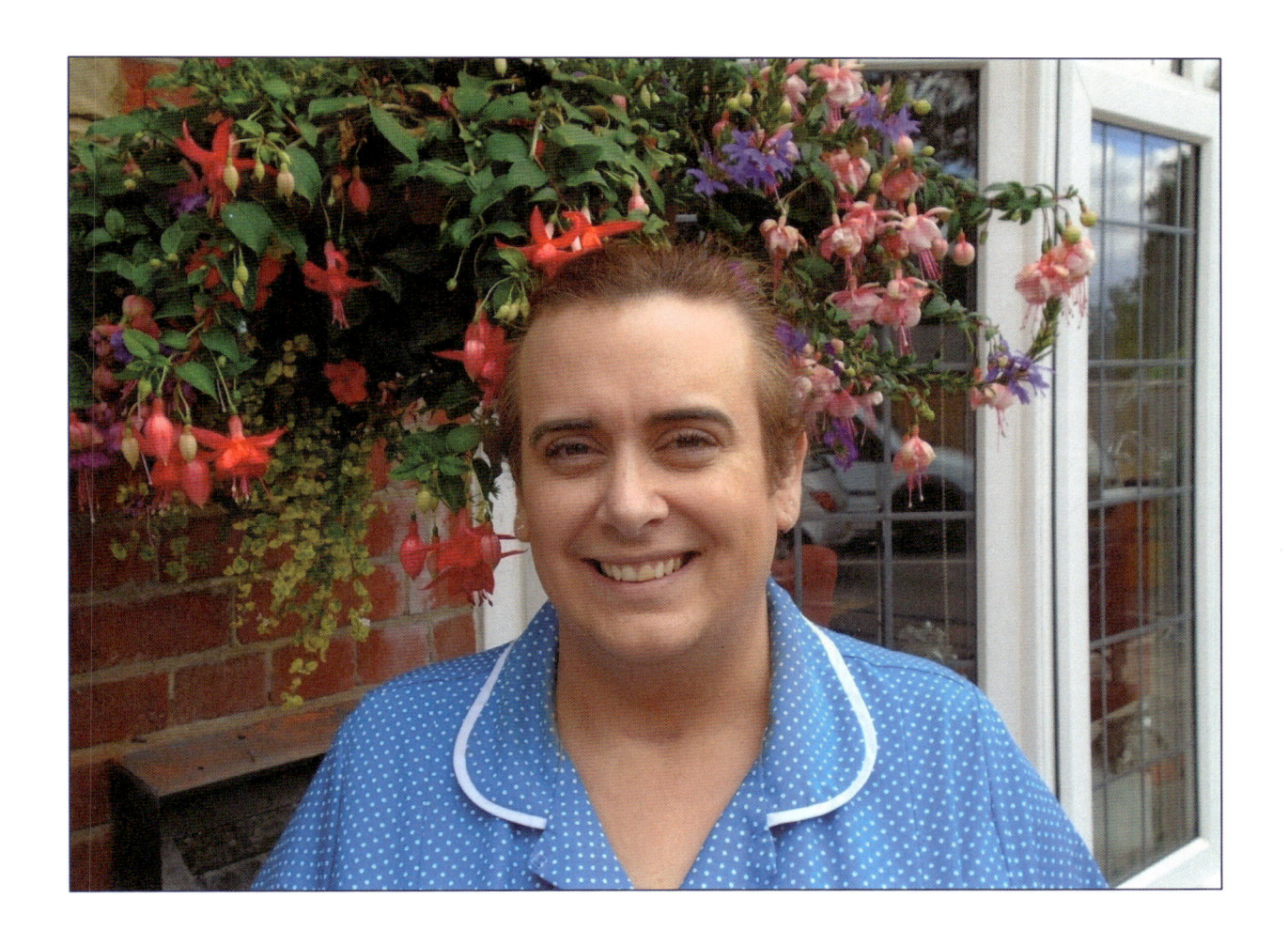

It is the carers who ultimately define the character of the establishment.

And so, the word 'care' is the focus and definition of what a Care Home should provide. Here is a little verse that may help to illustrate the concept.

> Come to me my little child
> Cried the Shepherd to his sheep
> I heard you calling in the wild
> Amid the valleys deep
>
> And rolling hills so cold and bare
> In Morning's early light
> But do not fear the shadows there
> That dance within your sight
>
> Come and feel my warm embrace
> And let your heart be free
> There can be no finer place
> On Earth for you and me
>
> Within this precious moment caught
> As time goes rushing by
> The beauty of a fleeting thought
> But never asking why
>
> Some things are just meant to be
> It was always so
> So come my child and be with me
> Together we shall go
>
> Walking by the mountain stream
> And listening to the sound
> Of all that has here ever been
> In nature all around
>
> Come and let me comfort you
> And hold you close and then
> We'll walk together, just we two
> And never stray again

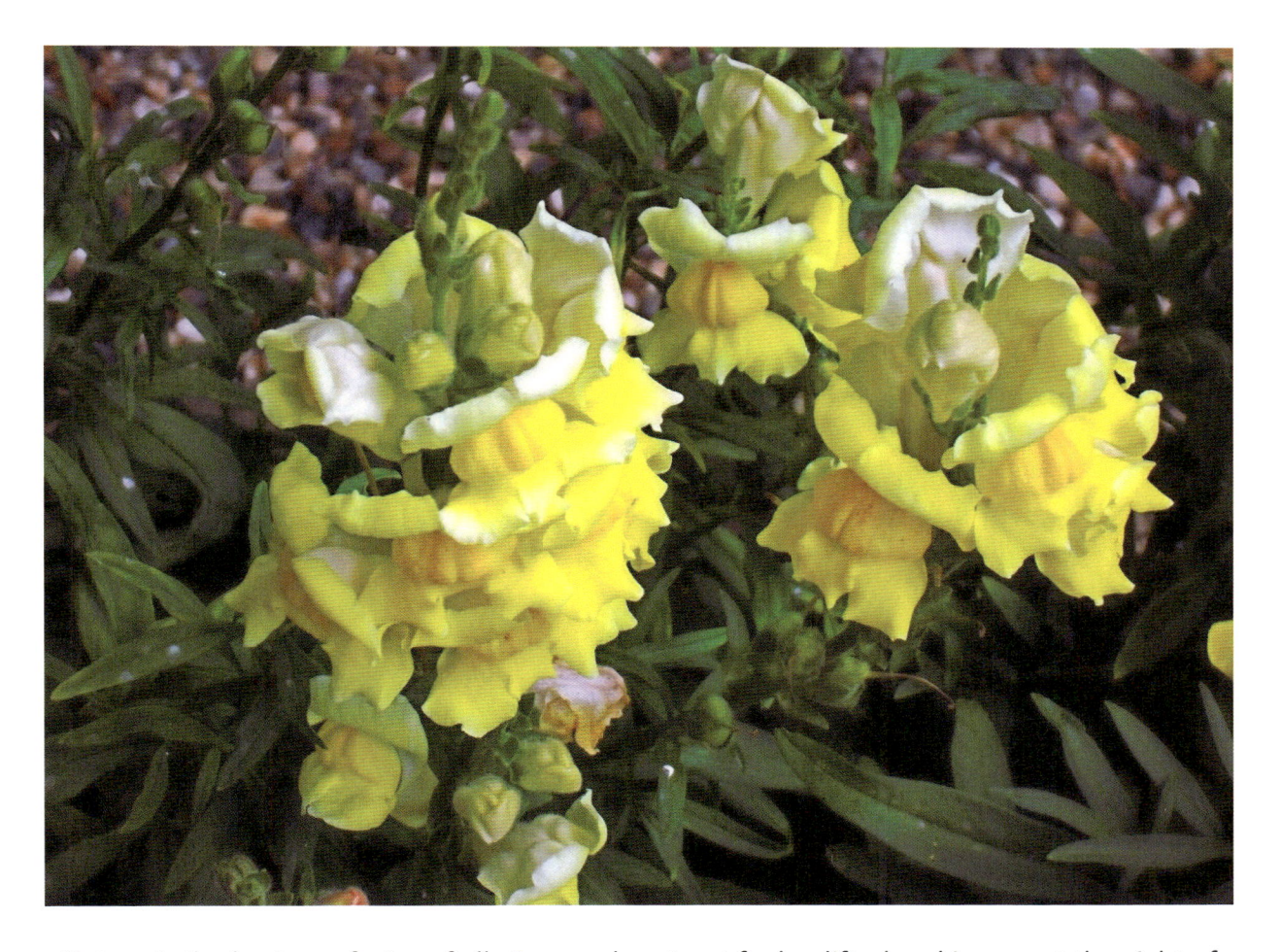

Nature is the best comforter of all. Can any heart not feel uplifted and joyous at the sight of such beauty, sitting there, all around?

6 The Residents

Probably, most people never think that they will end up in a Care Home. They rush through their lives, with the hustle bustle of their professional occupation and a social life which is modeled upon what they have been taught to be normal. Mostly, that means being a consumer of tourism, hobbies or some other activity which has a cost associated with it. In the modern world, more and more, everything is about money. There is a cost to everything and people are measured, not by character or kindness, but by how much money they make. We equate success in life purely with material worth and the trinkets of position and celebrity. Consequently, almost from birth, individuals are lured into this 'rat race' existence without taking the time to consider what is really important within our life's journey. There are exceptions of course, those whose lives revolve around kindness and understanding. Understanding of the world, of nature, of the arts, sciences and humanities. These individuals lead a fulfilled life, wherever they find themselves. Others never stop to think about such things, until, that is, they are hit by illness or infirmity in such a way that it is debilitating. And then, things move along quickly and, very soon, decisions must be made that we never expected would be the case.

Consequently, the residents of a Care Home may be something of a mixed bunch. Often, there will be a higher female than male count and, of course, there will be various stages of illness or infirmity. This all has to be managed by the staff.

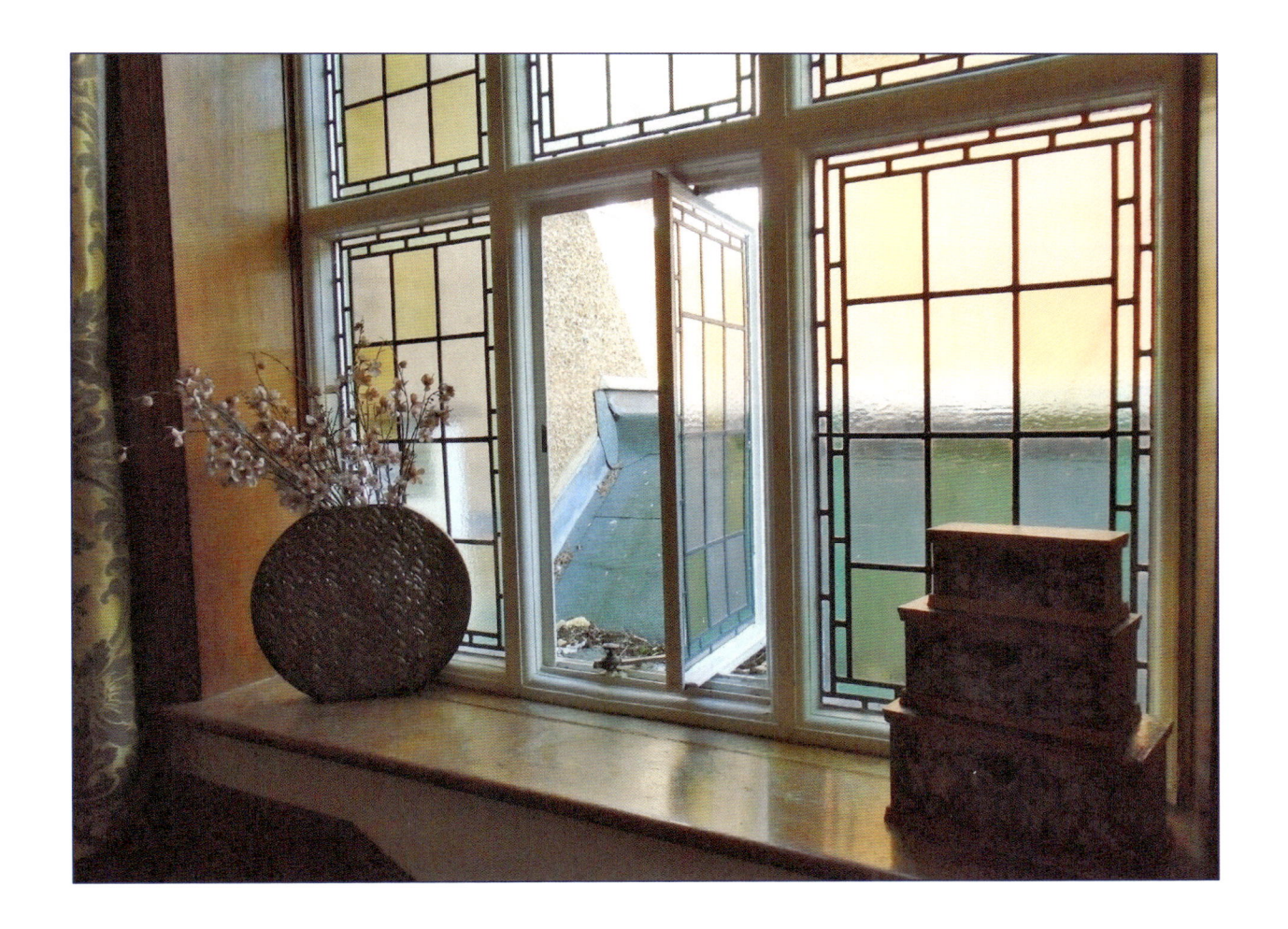

The windows of a Care Home are windows onto the outside world.

Many residents will remain mentally and physically active, while others might be more fragile and wheelchair bound, but still very aware of all that is going on around them and always ready for a chat or a joke. A common mistake is to assume that physical frailty must be reflected in mental capacity, but this is simply not the case. It is true that some residents may suffer with dementia, but even this condition has variations and does not mean that the sufferer is necessarily incapable of understanding. Other residents may be in a Care Home simply because they are suffering from a terminal illness, but might otherwise be OK and certainly capable of functioning in a normal manner. For these residents, the experience may be a little trying at times, as they hold on to their independence for as long as possible.

One thing that all residents have in common, is that they are human beings. They were all once somebody's beloved child who they bounced on their knee and watched grow up from infancy, through childhood and adolescence to adulthood. They all have a lifetime of rich experience upon which to ponder and, ironically, a great deal of interesting experience that they could share with the outside world, if anyone was interested. As an integral component of humanity, they deserve to be treated with respect and helped to maintain a dignified and meaningful existence, in spite of their condition. For some, this will be harder than for others, but the same principles of humanity apply.

Relatives are also affected of course and, for some, observing their loved one in such trying circumstances can be difficult. Indeed, relatives are as much a part of the overall picture as the residents themselves and must be treated with equal consideration. At Kilfillan House, relatives are always welcome and often participate in group activities.

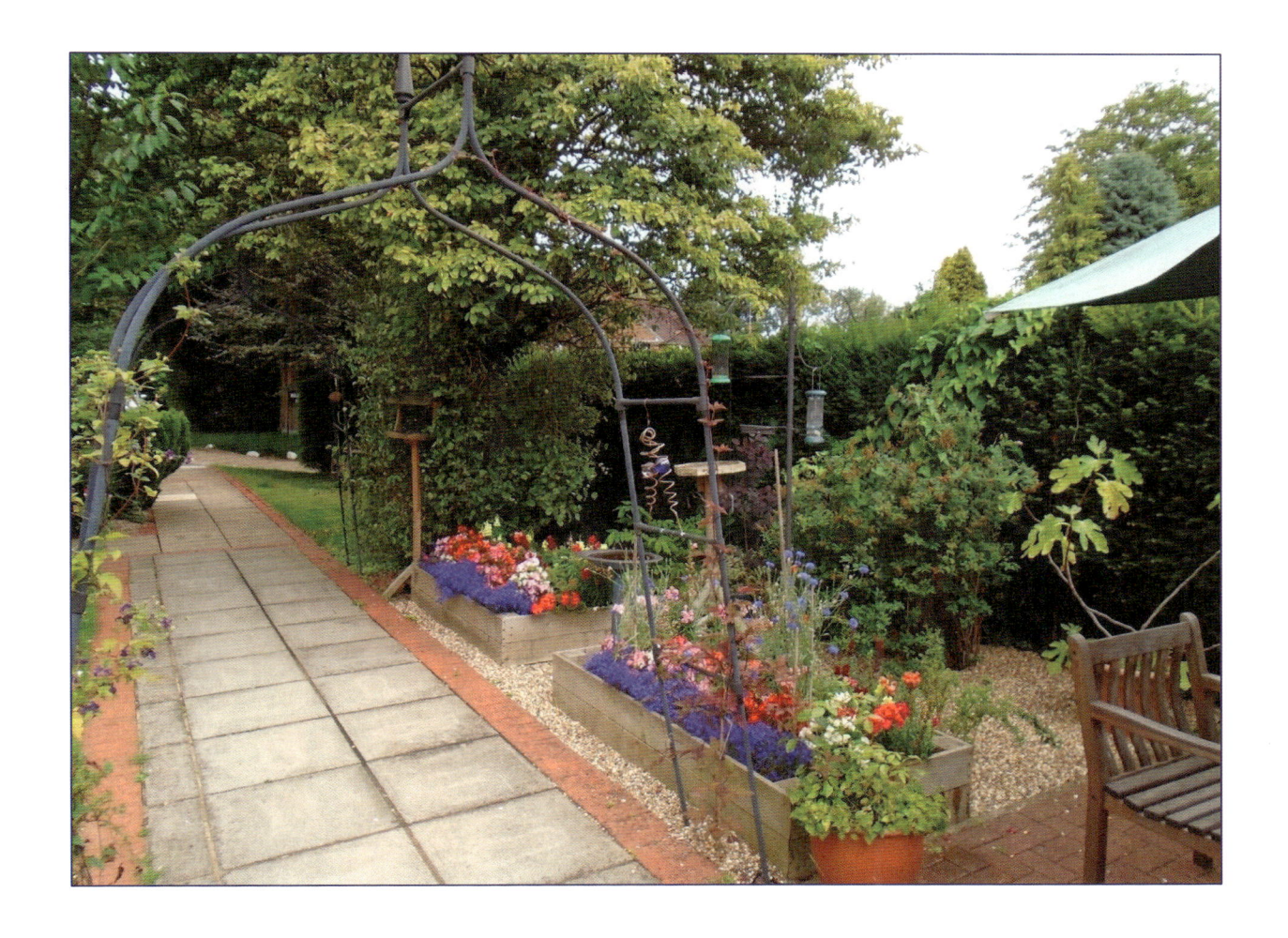

Everyone may enjoy the garden at Kilfillan House, residents and visitors alike.

6 Reflections

This book has provided an overview of a single Care Home, Kilfillan House, which happens to be situated at Berkhamsted in Hertfordshire. There are hundreds of such establishments, scattered across Britain, who all share a similar objective; to care for those who find themselves in need towards the end of their lives. Residents will be of various ages, some of them relatively young, perhaps in their early 60s, while many may be in their 80s or 90s. Caring for these individuals is a full time task and not for the feint hearted as carers will be faced with a number of quite challenging situations. Furthermore, there is the obvious emotional impact that such a specialist job implies. It is a job which will not suit everyone and good carers are a breed apart, combining endless patience with kindness and an empathy with those who are the recipients of their care. They are very special people and should be rewarded for their efforts to a greater degree than is currently the case. They also tend to work long shifts, making this quite a tiring occupation.

Duty nurses also work long shifts and, typically, will have upwards of twenty individuals to keep an eye on and for whom they must administer the correct medication. This is hard work. In addition, for certain conditions, like dementia for example, there exists a degree of unpredictability for which they must be prepared. Understanding, in detail, the particular condition of a large group of patients and being aware of how these conditions might advance and what to look for, is a significant and highly responsible task. They too should be properly rewarded for the important task that they perform.

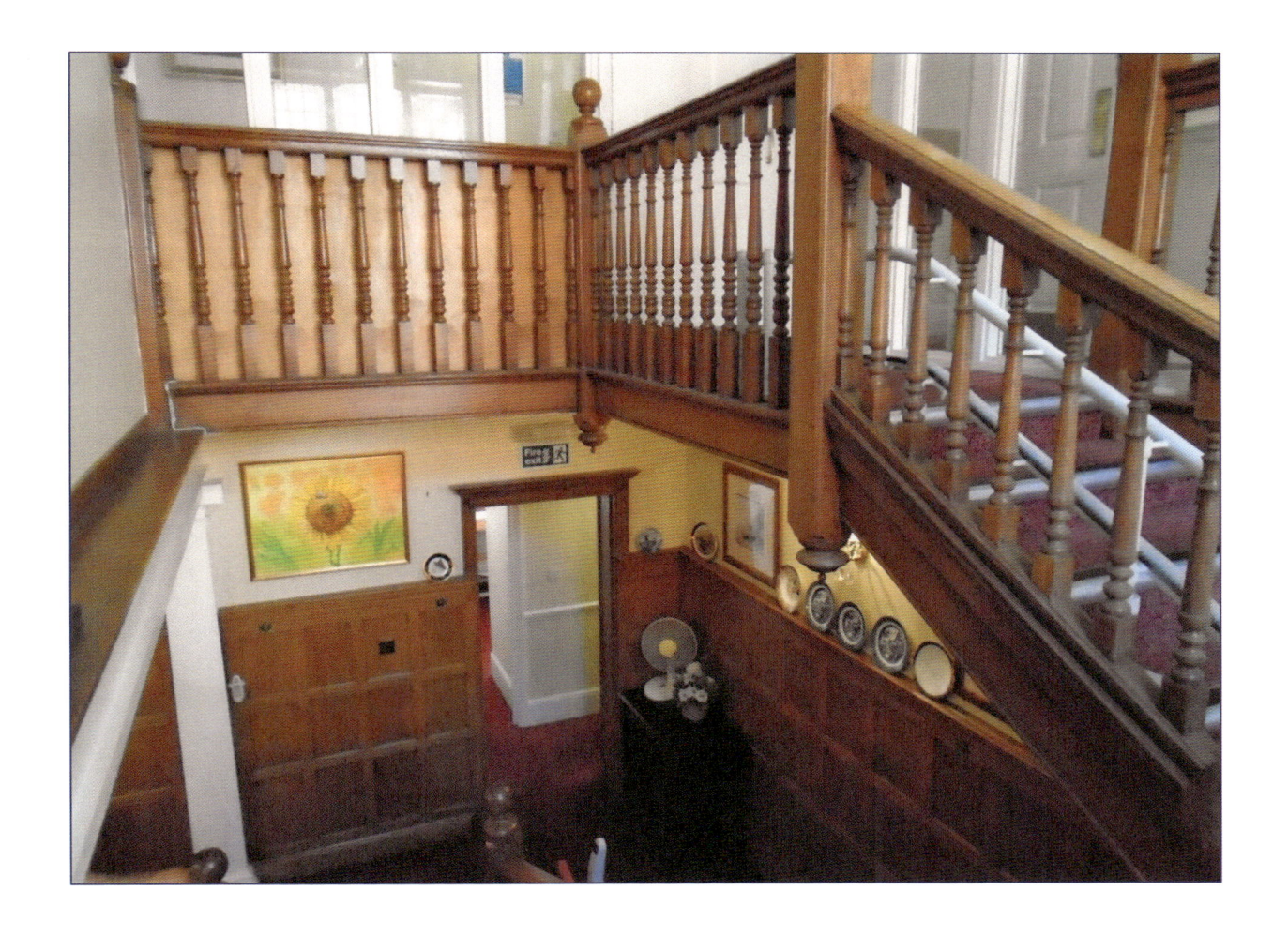

How many must have have trodden the stairs, up and down, at Kilfillan House over the years.

The unfortunate fact is that, in Britain, Care Homes are becoming over-subscribed as the burgeoning over population of our little island continues. Consequently, there are more people of every age group, including the elderly. This is entirely due to the short sightedness, or what some would call rank stupidity, of successive governments. The same is true at the other end of the age scale, where we are struggling to provide enough schools. Other social services are at breaking point, Doctor's Surgeries have started to block any new patients, and yet, the government continues to close down hospitals hand over fist, and remove support in many other areas for those in need. Consequently, this further exacerbates the Care Home shortage and places additional pressure on existing facilities.

Given the above, it is quite marvelous that the staff of Care Homes, such as Kilfillan House, respond positively and continue, even though under great strain, to provide a very high standard of care. This is due entirely to the personalities of all of those involved, from the practice manager, through the administrative staff, to the nurses and carers, who give so much of their time, and so much of their lives, devoted to such a task. If a similar situation existed within commerce, industry and government agencies, perhaps the world might be a better place.

And so, we need to support our Care Homes and to build more of them in order that those who have already given so much throughout their working lives, may be properly cared for when they most need that sort of help. Such provision is surely the hallmark of a civilised society, especially after several millennia of such civilisation throughout the evolution of humanity.

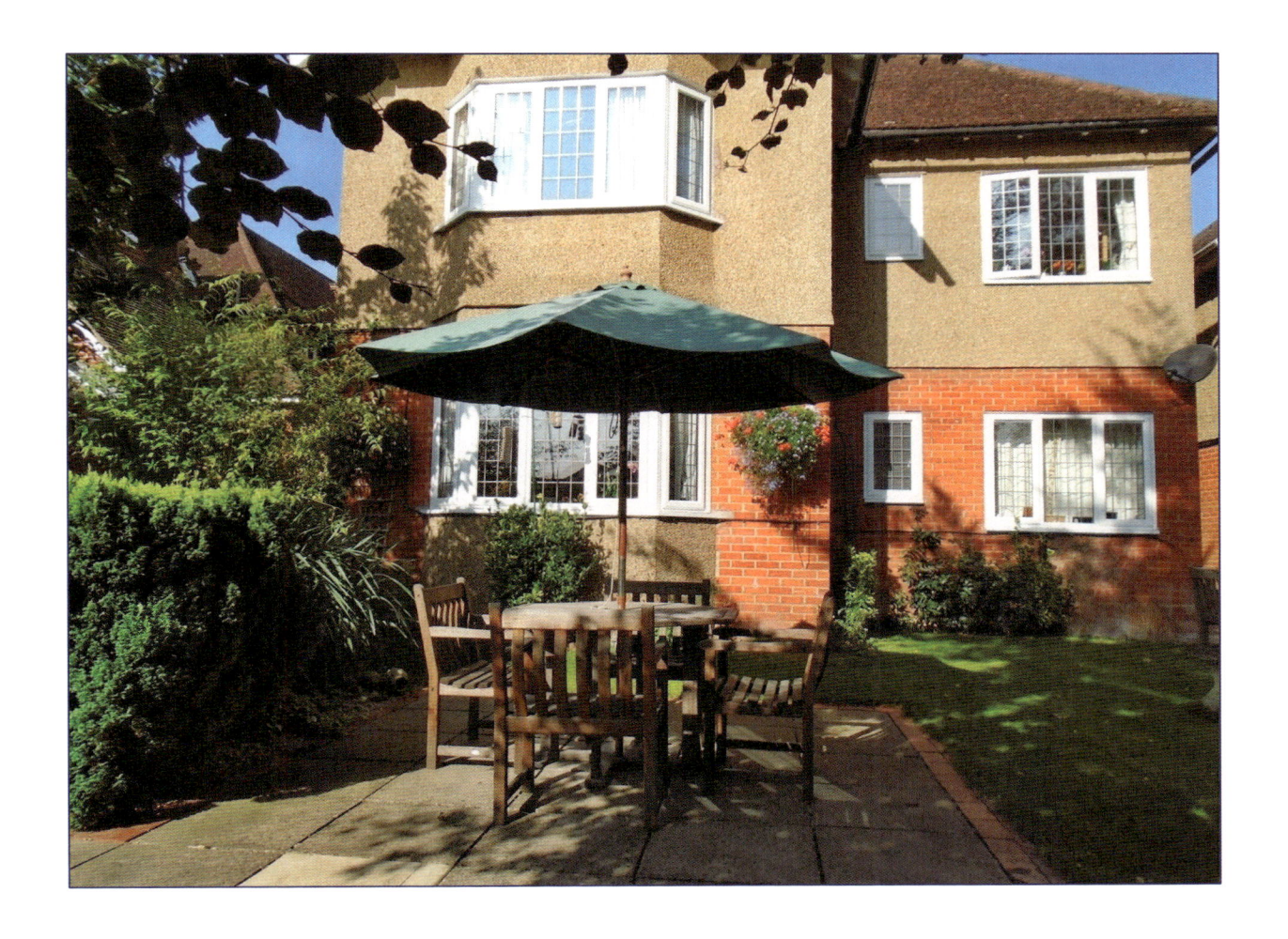

Part of the rear of Kilfillan House. A nice spot to enjoy the sunshine.

This book has provided a short overview of a particular Care Home, Kilfillan House, in order that the reader may better understand just how such an establishment functions. As such, it may prove invaluable to those facing the possibility of becoming resident within such a facility. However, perhaps the primary question that such an individual, or their close relative, might ask, I what is life actually like for a patient in such facility?

In this book, the terms 'patient' and 'resident' have been used interchangeably. Indeed, they both apply as the individuals concerned are both. They are residents in the sense that the Care Home becomes their home. The place where they live, receive visitors and enjoy the various activities available. They are also patients in the sense that they do need to be cared for from a medical perspective and their condition closely monitored.

I will use my own experience to describe a typical day in the life of a resident. Sometime between 07.00 and 07.30, the duty nurse will bring my morning medication. Shortly afterward, a carer will appear and ask me what I would like for breakfast. This is usually brought to my room between 07.30 and 07.45, and I will enjoy breakfast while listening to the radio. At around 08.00 I will telephone my wife and then have a shave and good wash, before getting dressed for the day. I might then go for a short walk, or perhaps sit in the conservatory for a while with one of my books. A carer will usually bring me a cup of tea and ask me if I am OK. As I have a mobility scooter, I may go for a ride into town or to the nearby woods, a pleasure that, sadly, few are able to enjoy. If the weather is agreeable, this is something which I really enjoy and will make the most of while I am still able. I park my scooter in a corner of the conservatory, from where it is easily navigated to the main road outside and from where I may decide where to go for a short run.

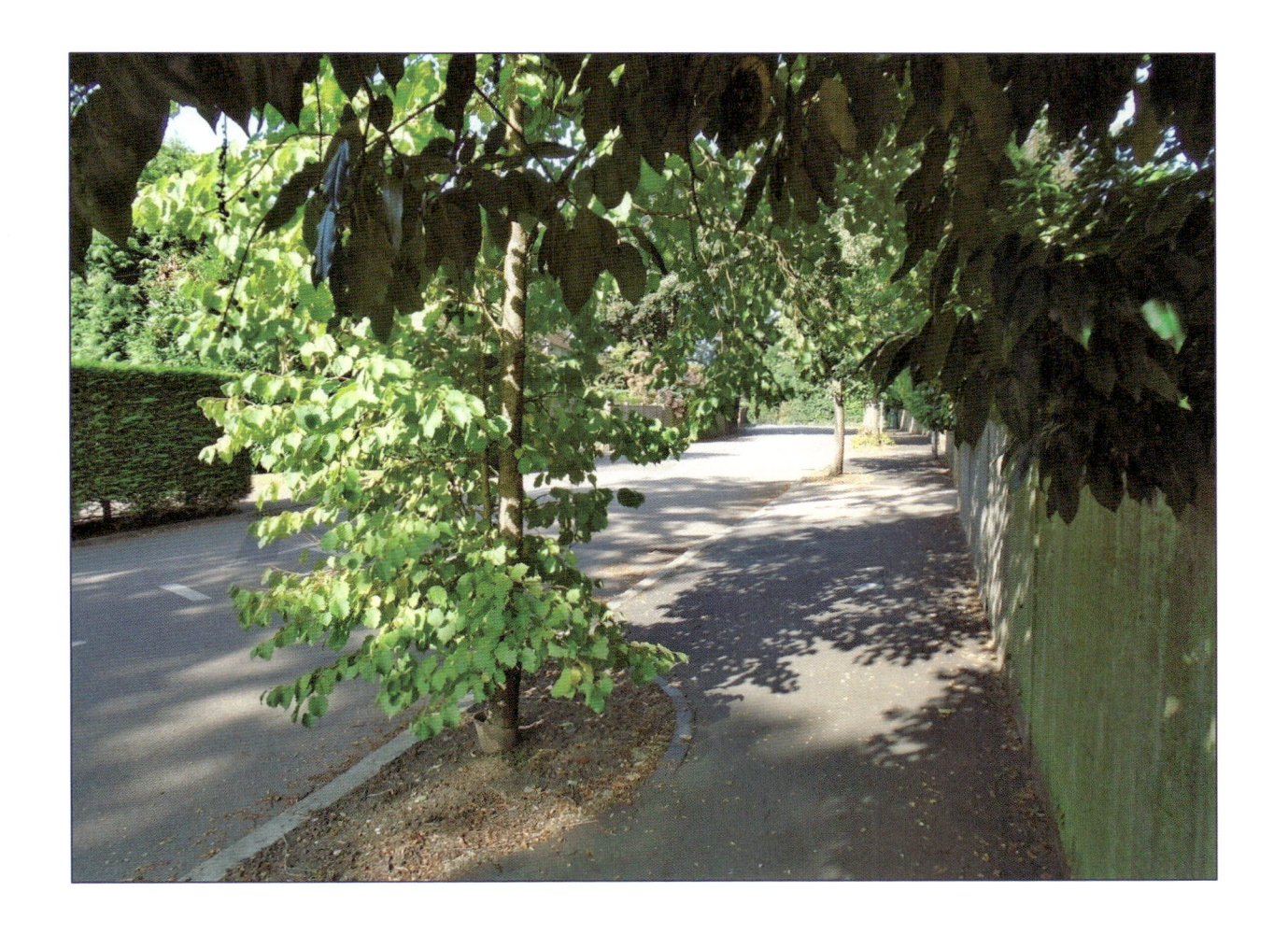

Graemesdyke Road, seen from the entrance to Kilfillan House.

At around 12.30 to 13.00, lunch is served, both in the dining room downstairs and in the resident's room if preferred. I usually take lunch in my room, together with my mid-day medication. There is always a choice of menu at lunch time and, if nothing on the menu appeals, then something will be prepared especially for the resident concerned. After lunch, and a nice cup of tea, residents typically congregate in the conservatory and the lounge, where, on most days, there is some activity or other. Maybe a quiz, or perhaps an external entertainer. The walls of Kilfillan have reverberated to a wide range of entertainment, from Ladies Choirs to Ukulele Bands and pretty much everything in between.

At 17.00, supper is served from a fixed menu which is well considered, usually with a tasty second course. At 18.00 I have more medication, after which I might read or listen to music in my room for a while. Or perhaps go out for a short walk. At 20.00 I have more medication, after which I shall amuse myself, often with some personal project in which I am engaged or, if I am feeling tired, perhaps I will watch one of my favourite films on DVD. At 22.00 I have my last medication of the day, by which time I am usually ready to turn in, unless I am engaged in answering email messages or some other activity. Finally, I shall go to bed, but the caring does not stop. Throughout the night, carers or nurse will gently open the door to check that everything is OK. If I am awake, we exchange greetings, otherwise it is comforting to know that such an activity is occurring.

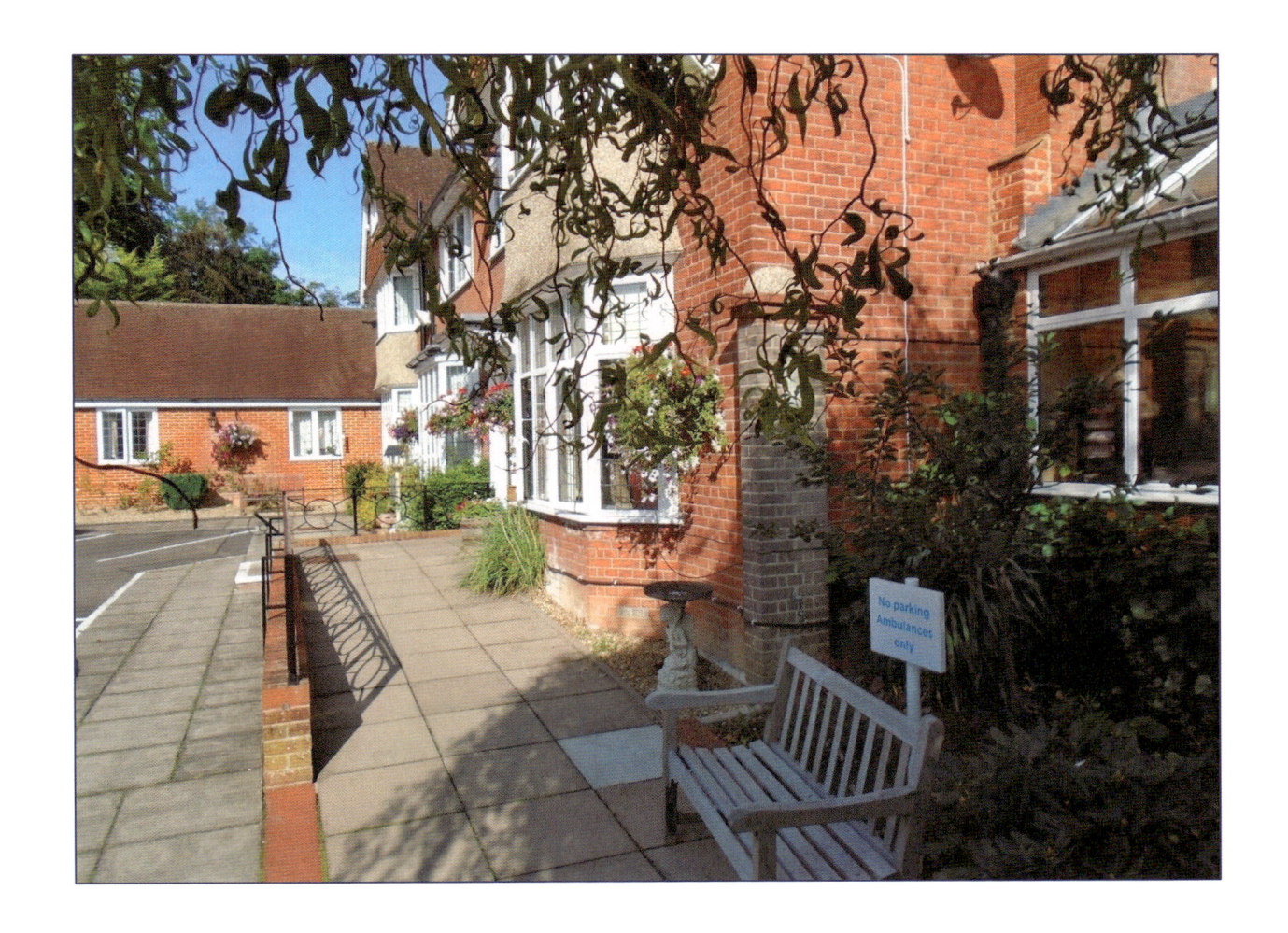

Another view of the front of Kilfillan House and the gentle slope to the front door.

Of course, the daily experience will be different for each resident. Those that are mobile will clearly have more options for taking a short walk and generally getting around. Those that are wheelchair bound may be taken to wherever they would most like to be. Often, they will congregate in the conservatory for a chat or to engage in some sort of group activity. Sometimes, they will stay in the lounge and watch television. They very much enjoy the entertainment that is provided regularly. Naturally, a few residents are completely bedbound and unable to participate in such things. Generally, these individuals will be very seriously ill and will require a great deal of attention from the staff. However, they all have televisions in their rooms if they wish to watch them, and so they are not completely bereft of entertainment.

Life in the Care Home is not unlike life at home, except that there are carers constantly on hand and the resident may be sure that they will receive their medication on time. This medication will be prescribed by their doctor, in consultation with the nurses at the Care Home and, very often, with specialist consultants, depending upon their particular illness or condition. This ensures that the patient is constantly monitored and may be provided with the best possible care at all times.

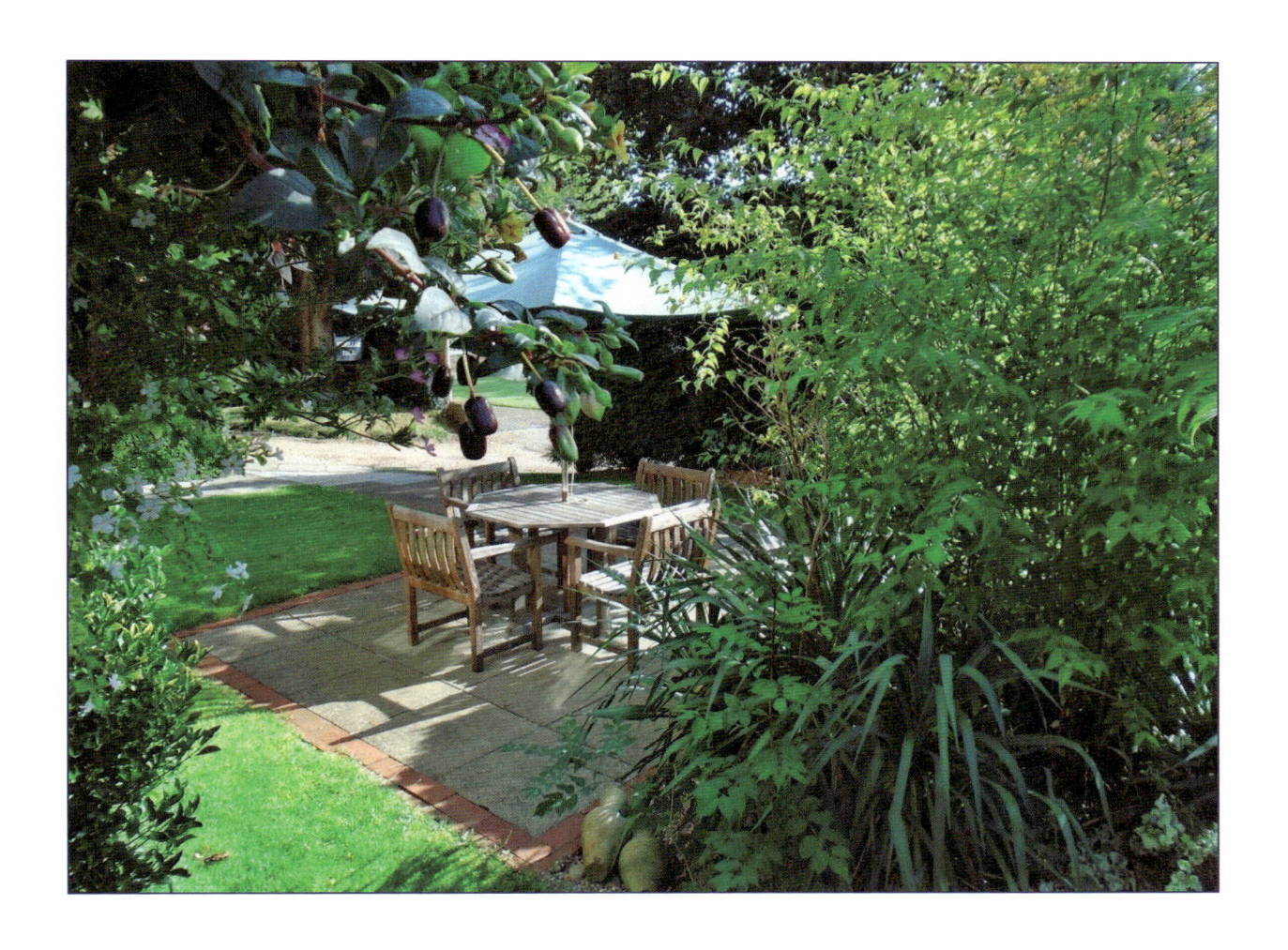

Life finds a way, all around Kilfillan House.

This book has provided a walk through the gardens and common areas of Kilfillan House, together with some discussion as to the functionality of a Care Home and this Care Home in particular. It has also provided a perspective on what it is like to be a resident in such an establishment. Perhaps this will be useful for those contemplating such a move. However, perhaps more than anything, the book has provided an insight into Kilfillan House itself as a Care Home. In particular, the staff who, day in and day out, work so diligently and so hard in order to care for the residents. Here, and on the next page, is a fitting little verse to celebrate these individuals.

Angels fly across the skies
At least, that's what we always thought
Rarely seen by human eyes
Just as we were always taught

But maybe that is not quite true
Perhaps sometimes they do descend
And settle down within our view
Just briefly, while they make amends

For all the heartache here beset
That comes and holds us in its grip
And all the things we do regret
All those moments we let slip

For angels walk upon this Earth
Of that, there truly is no doubt
Guiding us to all that's worth
Sharing with those all about

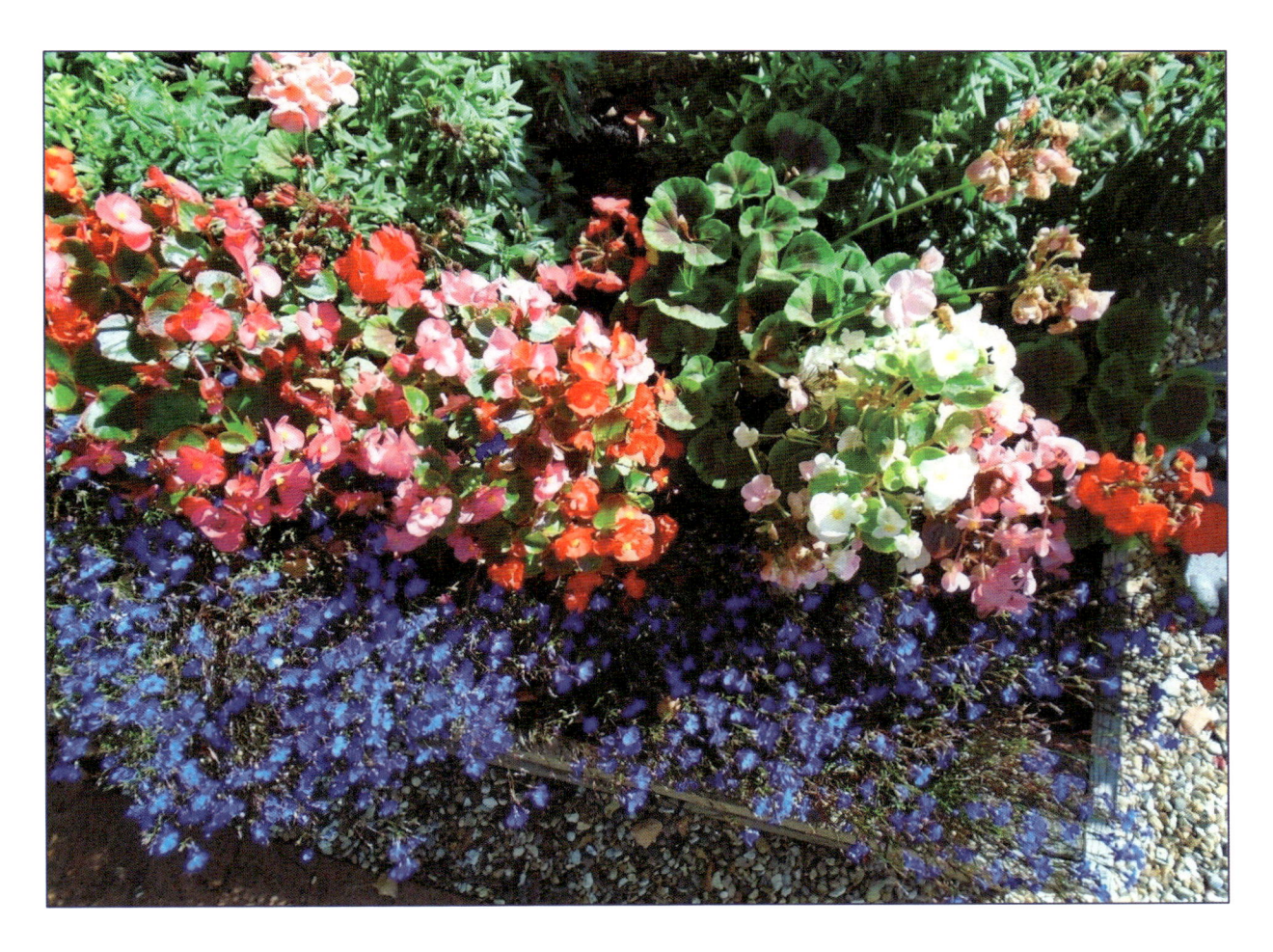

There is a splash of colour around every corner at Kilfillan House.

Love and kindness, friendship too
And all those good things in our hearts
Bringing hope to see us through
And helping us to make a start

To organize our own brief days
Along the lines that they have shown
Sharing in so many ways
The love within us that has grown

Throughout the times where we have been
So lucky on this path of life
And all the goodness we have seen
So rarely tainted there with strife

So watch out for those angels do
As they perform their kindly deeds
They're standing there right next to you
So let them sow their loving seeds

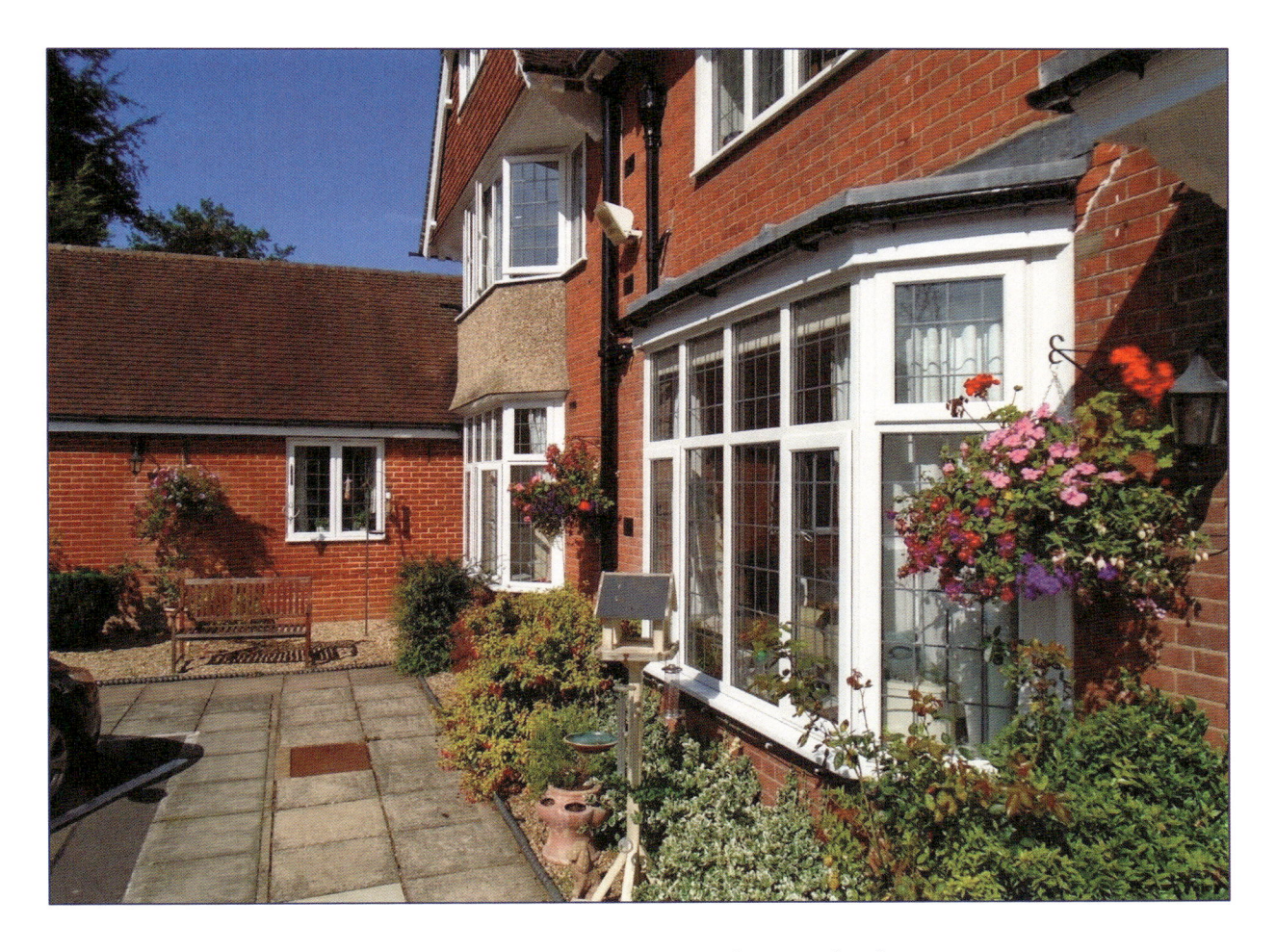

Baskets and shrubs add more colour at the front.

And now, I will insert a few blank pages in order for the reader to make their own notes, while we take a last stroll around the Kilfillan gardens. Thank you for reading this book. I do hope that it has brought you some pleasure.
J.A.

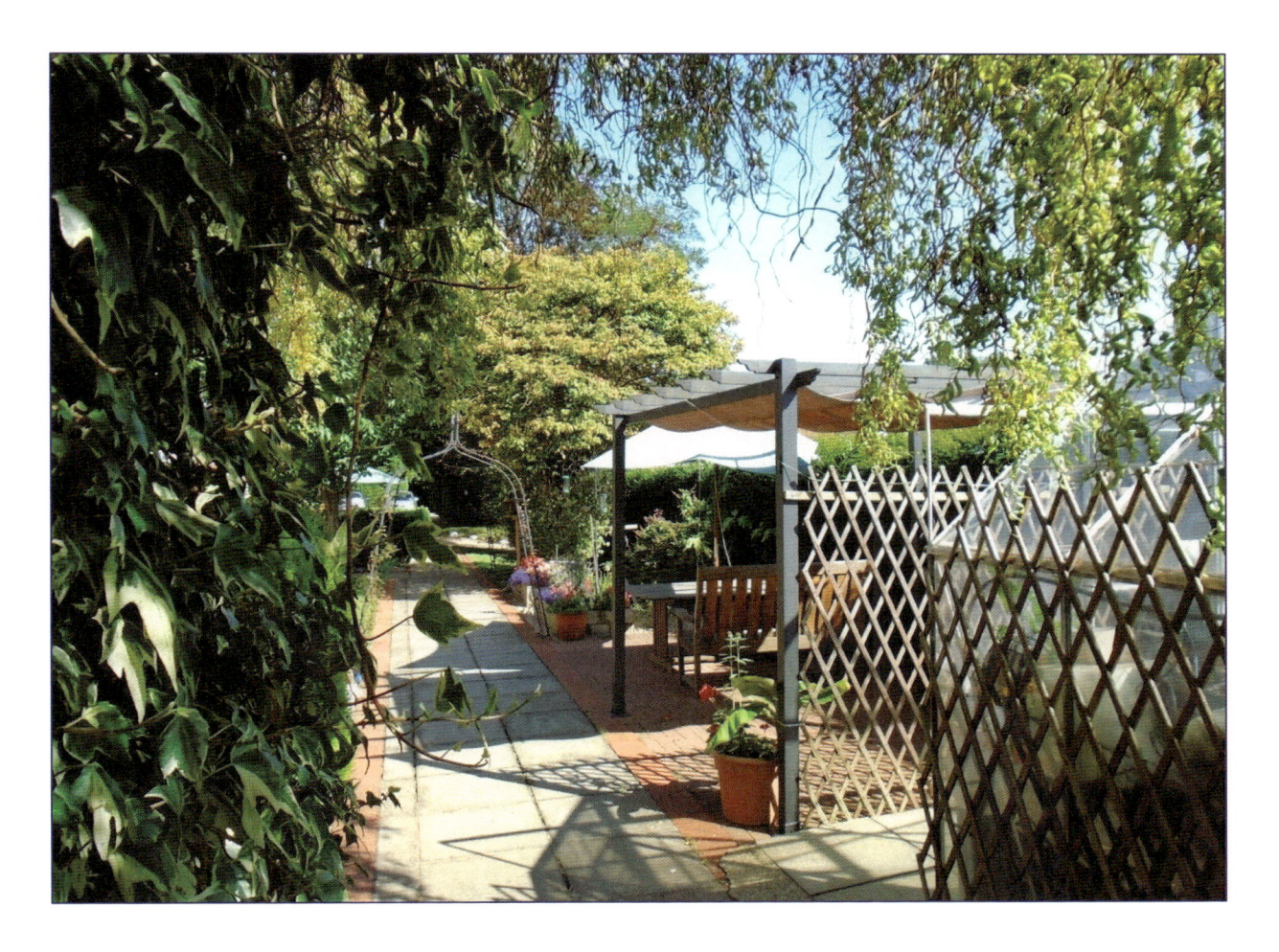

On the main path, passing the greenhouse on the right.

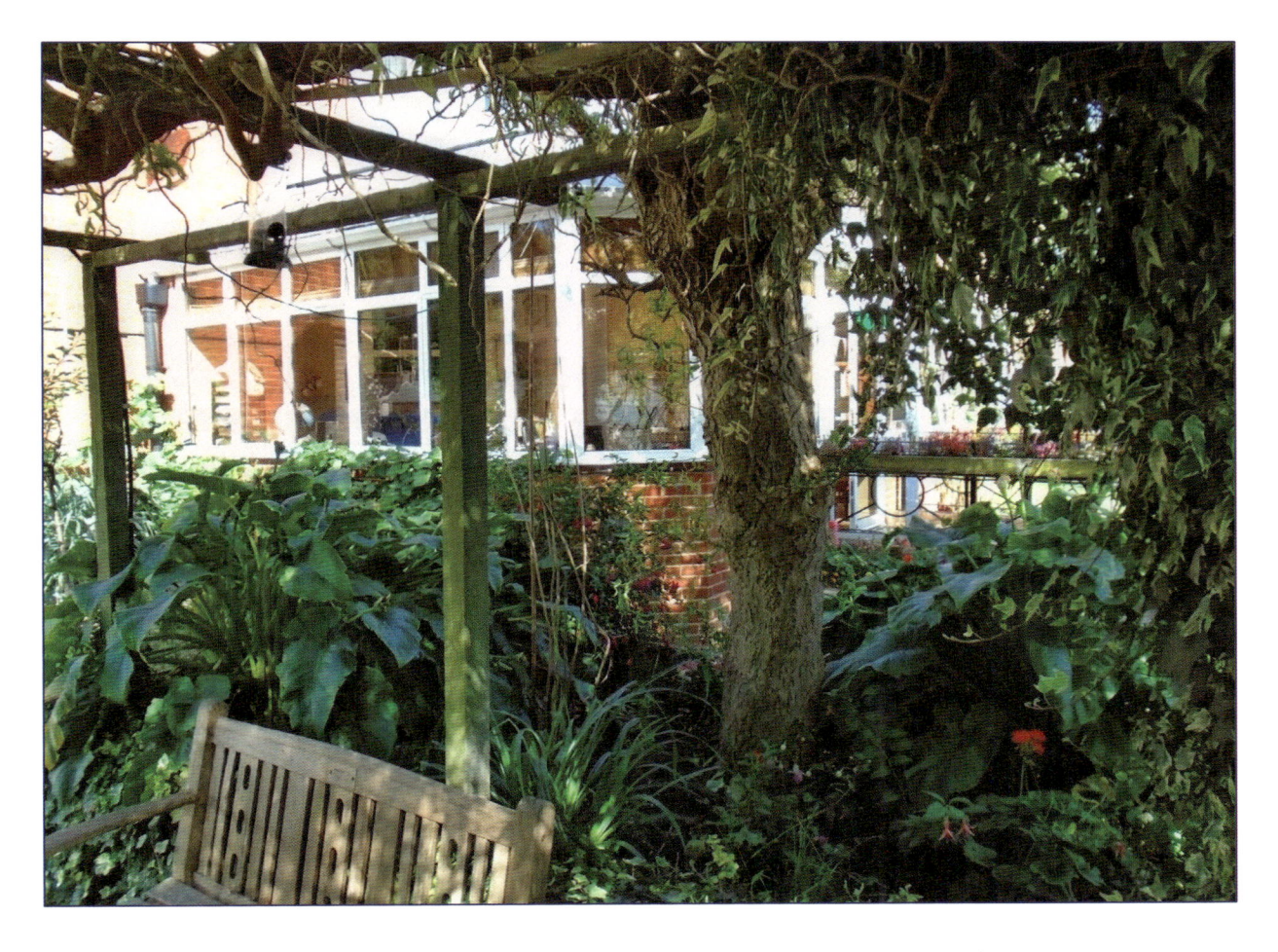

A jungle eye view of the house. Actually, this is a very pleasant place to sit.

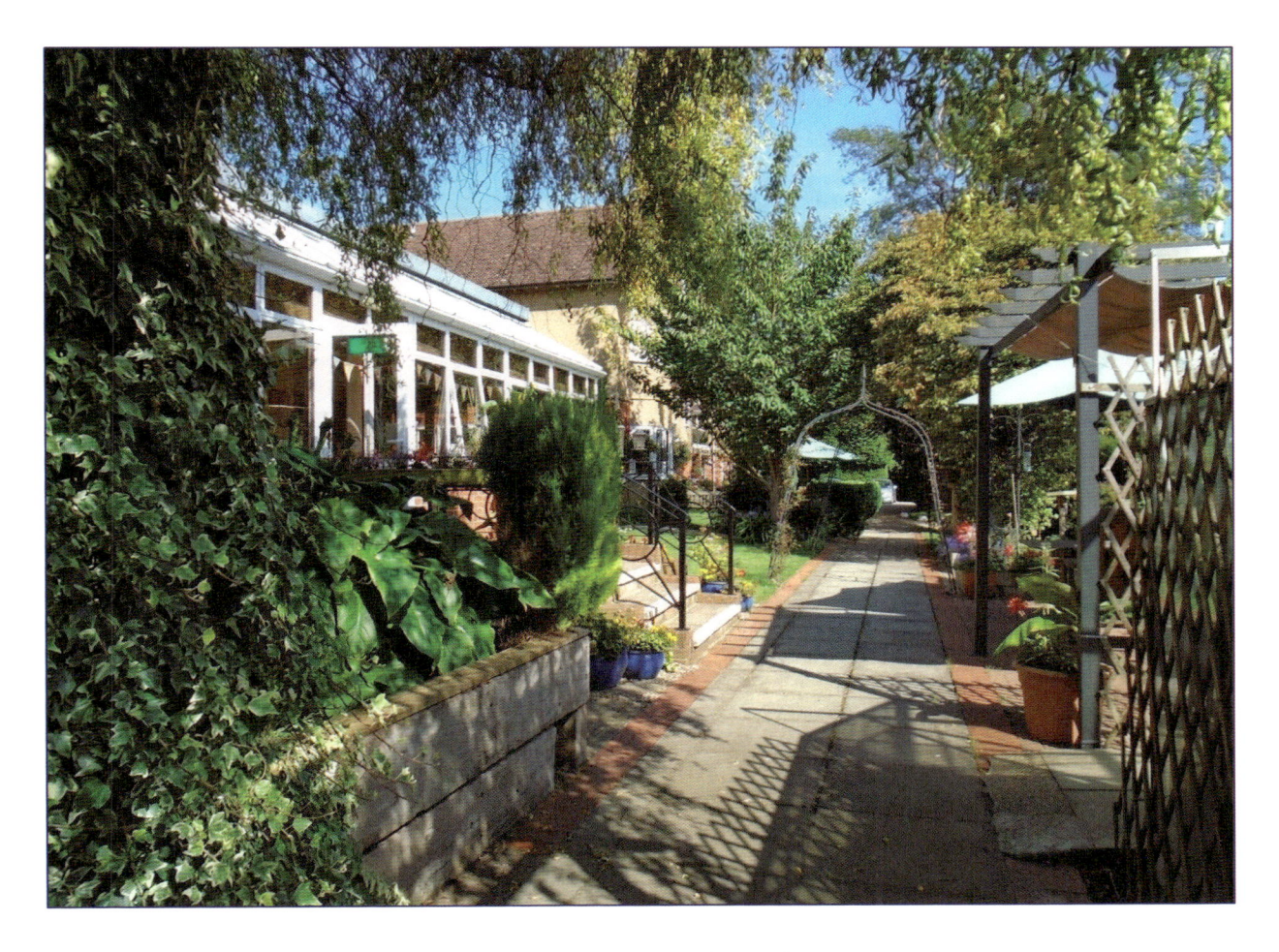

Approaching the conservatory from the main path.

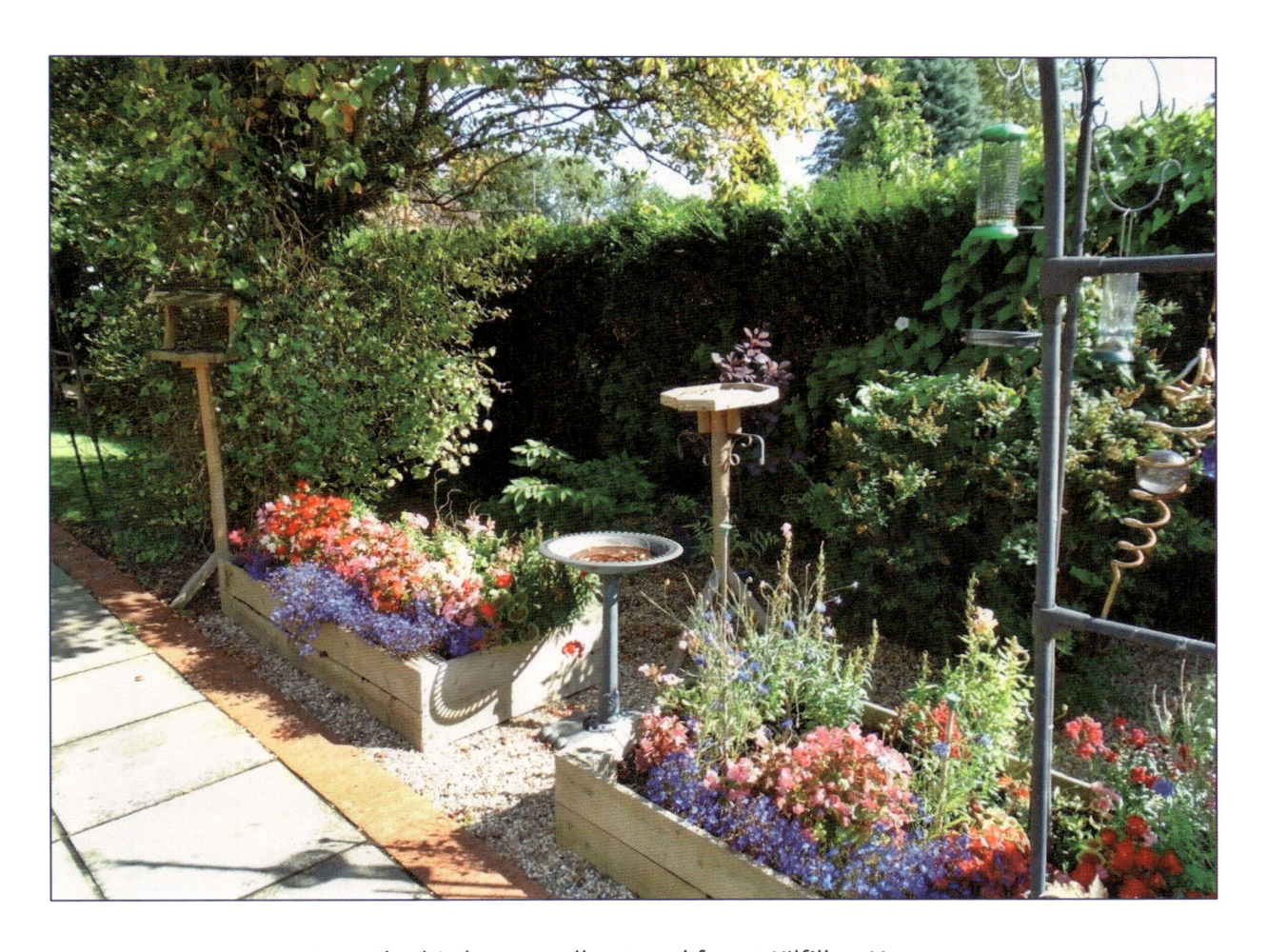

Even the birds are well catered for at Kilfillan House.

Thank you,
Au revoir

Made in the USA
Columbia, SC
28 August 2017